CAN'T CATCH A BREAK

CAN'T CATCH A
BREAK

GENDER, JAIL, DRUGS, AND THE LIMITS
OF PERSONAL RESPONSIBILITY

Susan Starr Sered and
Maureen Norton-Hawk

 UNIVERSITY OF CALIFORNIA PRESS

University of California Press, one of the most distinguished university presses in the United States, enriches lives around the world by advancing scholarship in the humanities, social sciences, and natural sciences. Its activities are supported by the UC Press Foundation and by philanthropic contributions from individuals and institutions. For more information, visit www.ucpress.edu.

University of California Press
Oakland, California

Parts of chapter 5 have appeared in "Suffering in an Age of Personal Responsibility," *Contexts* 13 (2014):38–43. Parts of chapter 6 have appeared in "Criminalized Women and Twelve Step Programs: Addressing Violations of the Law with a Spiritual Cure," in *Implicit Religion* 15, no. 1 (2012): 37–60; and "Whose Higher Power: Criminalized Women Confront the Twelve Steps," in *Feminist Criminology* 6, no. 4 (2011): 308–322. Parts of chapter 7 have appeared in "Mothering in the Shadow of the United States Correctional System," in *Mothering: Anthropological Perspectives*, ed. Michelle Walks and Naomi McPherson (Toronto, Ontario: Demeter Press, 2011), 293–306.

Library of Congress Cataloging-in-Publication Data

Sered, Susan Starr, author.
    Can't catch a break : gender, jail, drugs, and the limits of personal responsibility / Susan Starr Sered and Maureen Norton-Hawk.
        pages   cm
    Includes bibliographical references and index.
    ISBN 978-0-520-28278-0 (cloth : alk. paper)
    ISBN 978-0-520-28279-7 (pbk. : alk. paper)
    ISBN 978-0-520-95870-8 (e-book)
    1. Abused women—Massachusetts—Boston—Social conditions.   2. Female offenders—Massachusetts—Boston—Social conditions.   3. Women drug addicts—Massachusetts—Boston—Social conditions.
4. Responsibility—Social aspects—Massachusetts—Boston.   I. Norton-Hawk, Maureen, author.   II. Title.
    HQ1439.B7S47   2014
    3628.83'70974461—dc23   2014011744

Manufactured in the United States of America

23 22 21 20 19 18 17 16 15 14
10 9 8 7 6 5 4 3 2 1

In keeping with a commitment to support environmentally responsible and sustainable printing practices, UC Press has printed this book on Natures Natural, a fiber that contains 30% post-consumer waste and meets the minimum requirements of ANSI/NISO Z39.48-1992 (R 1997) (*Permanence of Paper*).

CONTENTS

ILLUSTRATIONS

TABLES

ACKNOWLEDGMENTS

Our names are on the cover of this book, but the real authors are the women who so generously shared their time, experiences, and conversations with us. Although they cannot be named here because of their vulnerable life and legal situations, this is their story. We have done our best to tell it faithfully.

We wish to thank the many caseworkers, therapists, nurses, doctors, public defenders, counselors, and advocates who help poor, marginalized, sick, and criminalized Americans. These valiant frontline workers opened doors for us as researchers and generously shared their observations and expertise with us. Special thanks to Gina Dixon for helping us stay in touch with some of the women during their most difficult times.

We thank Suffolk University for providing summer research grants as well as an encouraging and supportive work environment. We especially thank the members of the Suffolk University Sociology Department, who put up with our turning the office into a drop-in center. The Center for Women's Health and Human Rights at Suffolk University contributed funding and support to this project from the beginning to the end. We are particularly grateful to our colleagues Amy Agigian, Diane D'Souza, and Elana Stone. Funding also was provided by the Center for Crime and Justice Policy Research, Suffolk University.

Our warmest thanks to Thomas Patterson, who always made the women feel welcome when they came to see us at Suffolk University.

This research would have been impossible without the generosity of the Massachusetts Bay Transit Authority Transit Police. Their donation of mass-transit passes encouraged the project participants to maintain regular contact with us and compensated participants for the time they spent helping with the project.

Experts in a number of fields generously vetted chapters for us. We wish to thank our colleague James Ptacek for help with chapter 1, "Joey Spit on Me." His expertise in the field of intimate partner violence was invaluable. George Lipsitz of the Department of Black Studies (University of California, Santa Barbara) and our Suffolk colleague Averil Clarke helped us understand intersections of race, gender, and class for chapter 3, "The Little Rock of the North." Dr. Jeffrey Baxter, addiction consultant for the Massachusetts Department of Corrections and professor in the Department of Family Medicine and Community Health at the University of Massachusetts Medical School graciously read and critiqued chapter 4, "Suffer the Women: Pain and Perfection in a Medicalized World," and shared with us his vast experience working with addicts. Jesse Begenyi of the Massachusetts Transgender Political Coalition encouraged us to feature "Ginger," and pointed out to us ways in which her experiences are similar and different from those of other transwomen. Our dear friend Janet Yassen, longtime anti-violence advocate, therapist, and crisis services coordinator for the Victims of Violence program at Cambridge Hospital, shared her expertise and experience with us for chapter 5, "'It's All in My Head.'" Our colleague Erika Kates, founder of the Massachusetts Women's Justice Network, and our Suffolk colleague Erika Gebo provided expert assistance with chapter 8, "Gender, Drugs, and Jail." We appreciate their collegiality, dedication, encouragement, and critical thinking about these complex issues.

We are fortunate to have worked with Maura Roessner at the University of California Press. Her unflagging enthusiasm for the project and her ability to help us sort out the forest from the trees are extraordinary. And we especially thank Steven Baker, whose guidance both in style and in substance went way beyond the duties of copyediting.

We have also been blessed with an incredible team of dedicated research assistants at Suffolk University. Each has contributed to this project in countless valuable ways: Annie Duong, Christina Tucciarone, Ellesse Akre, Rachel Bieu, Andrea Blasdale, Cathryn Duff-Still, Torrey Giaquinta, Joanna Prager, Jen Sturman, Ashley Terhune, and Nicole Usher. Thank you!

In addition to the Suffolk team, Susan appreciates the ongoing support, encouragement, and intellectual involvement of two other teams. Thank you to my Rosh Hodesh sisters: Debra Cash (writer extraordinaire), Julie Arnow, Ronnie Levin, Stephanie Loo, Shosh Schnur, and Vivian Troen. Thank you and all my love to my family: Yishai, Barak, Yoav, Asher, Shifra, Dad, and Barbara. And a special wag to Thorfinn and to Scout, who may not have contributed much intellectually to the project but certainly helped Susan stay calm and upbeat during some of the more harrowing moments.

We have received support and encouragement from Massachusetts state representative Kay Khan and from Lisa Rosenfeld, counsel and legislative director of the Joint Committee on Children, Families, and Persons with Disabilities (Massachusetts). In return, we offer them this book as a tool for legislative initiatives and advocacy on behalf of all who struggle with poverty, illness, and violence.

Introduction

When Francesca came bursting onto the scene at the drop-in center for poor and homeless women, she brought a spark of energy into the circle of worn-out faces and worn-down bodies, women slumped in armchairs, nodding off while watching *The Jerry Springer Show* and waiting for the shelters to reopen at 4:00. Outspoken, energetic, and full of plans, Francesca declared how terrible it is that Boston's "Mayor Menino stands by while so many people have to live on the street." With a few tosses of her long, auburn hair, she shared her dream of opening and running a facility that "welcomes everyone." Five minutes later she swept out the door into the August heat with a promise to "buy Pepsi for everybody." Ginger resumed her desultory search through a pile of donated toiletries, Elizabeth continued weeping into a handful of tissues, and Vanessa went back to scratching her arm and poking around in the trash in hopes of finding a cigarette stub long enough to take outside and light up.

A week later Francesca returned to the women's center. Flashing her new turquoise acrylic nail extensions, she pulled a sequined minidress and a pair of 1960s style go-go boots out of a bag. With the recession that began in 2007 having shut down employment opportunities for undereducated and unskilled workers, she had taken one of the few jobs she could get—waitressing and dancing at a local strip club. Thrilled with the clothes as well as the admiration from male patrons, she nevertheless was adamant that she would not have sex with the customers—she wouldn't even let them kiss her on the cheek. But by late fall the situation became tense. At the club, she said, "the owners expect the girls to have sex for money." As time went on, she began going out on "dates" and drinking more heavily as a way to put up with the pressures of the men at the club. "It is starting to get out of control," Francesca confessed.

Francesca had always loved dancing, but the long shifts at the club started to catch up with her. One night her knee gave out. Unable to go on dancing, she was fired on the spot. Initiating what would become a routine for the next five years, Francesca called us. We picked her up a block away from the club and drove her to the apartment of her old boyfriend who was willing to let her stay with him at night but would not give her a key or allow her to stay in the apartment by herself during the day.

Now a regular at the women's drop-in center, she tried to summon up her usual "I don't take crap from anyone" style, but began to confide to us that she felt afraid and vulnerable. "All I do is walk around all day—I have no place to go." Her arthritis had become increasingly painful (the joints in her fingers looked miserably swollen), and she said, "I have a pain in my throat that my doctor thinks might be throat cancer. My father died of cancer." Often on the verge of tears, she even considered suicide. "I just can't catch a break anywhere."

UNDER SIEGE: WOMEN IN AN UNFORGIVING WORLD

Several years before meeting Francesca, we traveled from Boston to northern Idaho and from the Mississippi Delta through the midwestern Rust Belt to southern Texas, speaking with working Americans caught in spirals of low-wage jobs, chronic illness, inadequate access to health care, visibly stigmatizing conditions (such as rotted teeth), and diminishing employment opportunities. At the time, we saw ourselves as cartographers mapping the portals into a vortex that seemed to draw in increasing numbers of Americans. Our mission was to understand how and why people who strive to "do the right thing" in terms of work and family find themselves barely scraping by (Sered & Fernandopulle 2005). Our concerns were well grounded in the statistics: nearly 4 million Americans work for hourly wages at or below the federal minimum of $7.25 an hour (Bureau of Labor Statistics 2013); nearly one out of two American adults live with at least one chronic illness (NCCDPHP 2009), with one-quarter of these men and women experiencing significant impairment in daily activities; and close to 30 percent of working-age adults with disabilities are impoverished (Anderson 2010).

As we said good-bye to the people we met on our journeys, we found ourselves worrying about their futures. In our imaginations we visualized further deterioration in health, leading to unemployability; homelessness; the management of pain and fatigue with Percocet, crystal meth, tobacco, and other drugs; involvement with police and courts; and even premature death. We began to wonder if we were witnessing the formation of an American caste of the ill and afflicted, and we asked ourselves where we might go to learn more about the lives and deaths of Americans stuck in conditions of illness and poverty.

Reports by experts in public health and criminology provided clues. America houses substantial numbers of ill and impoverished people inside prisons. According to statistics provided by the U.S. Department of Justice, 84 percent of inmates earned less than $2,000 a month, and 59 percent earned less than $1,000 a month, before they were incarcerated (James 2002). Over half of the incarcerated population have a mental health issue (James & Glaze 2006); at least 40 percent suffer from chronic illness (Cecere 2009); and about one-third have a significant hearing impairment (Vernon 1995). In addition to mental health challenges, inmates have higher rates of hypertension, myocardial infarction, asthma, arthritis, cervical cancer, urinary tract infections, chronic headaches, tuberculosis, and hepatitis than Americans in the general population (Massoglia 2008b).[1] Unhealthy prison conditions, coupled with the poor employment prospects facing ex-offenders (criminal records are easily accessed by potential employers), only partly explain the substandard health profile of Americans involved with the correctional system. Americans entering prison are already significantly sicker and poorer than other Americans (Wilper et al. 2009; Schnittker, Massoglia, & Uggen 2012).

In the nation with the highest incarceration rate in the world (753 prisoners for every 100,000 people; Schmitt, Warner, & Gupta 2010), approximately 2.2 million people are currently in America's prisons and jails, and around 7 million Americans are under some form of correctional supervision (Glaze & Herberman 2012). This is not an outlying minority; it is a substantial part of the American population. *Have prisons become the way that America deals with human suffering?*

Embedded in these grim statistics one group stood out to us. An estimated 70 percent of women drawn into the correctional system have experienced physical or sexual violence at some point in their lives (Chesney-Lind & Pasko

2004; McDaniels-Wilson & Belknap 2008; Bloom, Owen, & Covington 2004). Women prisoners have higher rates of HIV infection and other sexually transmitted diseases than male inmates, have higher rates of drug-use disorder, and are in greater need of mental health services (Arriola, Braithwaite, & Newkirk, 2006; Binswanger, Krueger, & Steiner 2009). Three-quarters of criminalized women live with chronic physical or mental impairments, or both, and *women prisoners are three times more likely than women in the general population to report poor physical and mental health* (James & Glaze 2006; LaVene et al. 2003). And while far more men than women are incarcerated, throughout the last two decades of the twentieth century and into the twenty-first, the rate of incarceration of women has increased more rapidly than the rate of incarceration of men (Heimer et al. 2012).

During the spring and summer of 2008, we set out to understand the lives of women who have experienced incarceration. Although we had seen the statistics showing that women who enter the correctional system are likely to have suffered rape, poverty, and serious illnesses, nothing had prepared us for the relentless afflictions plaguing the residents we were getting to know at a Boston halfway house for women on parole and at a nearby drop-in center for poor and homeless women.

Forty-seven of the women we met that spring and summer agreed to join us in a project that would follow their experiences for five years. Their average age in 2008 was thirty-six. The majority of the women were white (reflecting the demographics of Massachusetts). Most began their lives in working-class families. Many had been sexually abused as children. Nearly all had witnessed their mothers being beaten or verbally abused by husbands or boyfriends. Often they attributed their adult drug or alcohol use to these childhood experiences of violence. A few remembered pleasant childhoods with strong and positive family relations, but had found their lives spiraling downward as adults when their parents died and they could not afford to keep up with the rent or mortgage payments. Several women had become addicts through prescribed pain or anxiety medication in the wake of an illness, injury, or unsuccessful medical procedure. In their twenties most scraped by in the unstable occupational sectors of the working poor, such as food service and nursing homes. They raised their young children with sporadic financial contributions from male partners and with public assistance. Poor health eventually made it impossible for nearly all of these women to hold down jobs, leading to homelessness and vulnerability to exploitation and violence.

All of the women had been incarcerated, typically for a few months at a time and typically for prostitution, shoplifting, public drunkenness, possession of small amounts of drugs, involvement as accessories to a crime committed by a boyfriend or husband, or—most frequently—violation of the terms of probation or parole associated with a prior minor charge (in other words, the original charge had not been deemed sufficiently serious to require incarceration). For many of the women incarceration had led to loss of custody or contact with their children. Coming out of prison with their children gone, no money, and no home, they became ever more dependent upon public services, men, and the underground economy.

We were privileged to spend time with the Boston women in a variety of settings. Throughout the five years of the study, we tried to meet with each woman at least once a month for an informal chat, and at three-month intervals for a longer, more structured conversation regarding housing, money, jobs, family, relationships, and health since the previous conversation. As the women came to know us, we accompanied them to numerous court hearings, medical appointments, parties, shopping trips, christenings, weddings, birthdays, hospital stays, and program graduations. We also saw the women when we spent time at the various parks and drop-in centers they frequented. Of the forty-seven women who initially joined the project, thirty-two have remained in touch with us. Because most of the women did not have a permanent address or regular telephone service, keeping in contact was an enormous challenge that on many occasions we failed to overcome. Suffolk University's location afforded us a major advantage, as the campus is situated a block or so from the Boston Common, a large park where many homeless, unemployed, and marginalized Bostonians spend their days. Many of the women still like stopping by our office for a chat, a cup of coffee, or simply a quiet place to sit.

Throughout the study, we focused on the perceptions and viewpoints of the project women. We politely listened to opinions expressed by family members and by the many professionals with whom the women interact, but our commitment throughout has been to understand, to the best of our ability, how criminalized and marginalized women move through and interpret the world around them. Their stories emerged bit by bit over time. Often we didn't hear what we suspect is a core story until several years into the project, and even today we hear different versions of the same story and we witness unexpected interactions with friends, family, caseworkers, and correctional staff.

We took on this project with the expansive goal of understanding why so many Americans remain in circumstances that cause them to suffer. Our aim was not to test any particular hypothesis or probe a particular issue, but to gain a holistic appreciation of the experiences of this community of women over an extended period of time. The five-year span of the project allowed us to grow with the project women. We have developed significant relationships with at least some of them and have been with these women as their lives have changed and changed again. For several, their relationship with us became one of the longest-lasting and most stable ever experienced. For others, the incentive we provided (typically a monthly mass-transit pass) was the sole motivation for participating in the project. Several women said that they stuck with us because they were determined to finish one thing in their lives. A few made a point of telling us about problems that they wished us to pass along to the mayor, the courts, the governor, or the president, and we take that mandate seriously.

Every step of the way we have felt honored that people who have so much going on in their lives have been willing to take time to stay in touch with us and, often, to open their hearts and families to us. As social scientists we entered this project with the rather narrow goal of observing and recording what we observed; we believed in the accepted research methods of our disciplines—sociology and anthropology—and we felt a professional obligation to minimize our own impact on the community we had chosen to study (the "ethnographic field"). Over the years, we have come to see that this stance constitutes passive acceptance of a status quo that actively harms the women who have trusted us with their lives and their stories. This book, as well as our ongoing advocacy work, represents our commitment both to scholarship and to activism.

More about the project and the project participants can be found in the appendix at the end of the book.

NO HAPPY ENDINGS

When we first visited the halfway house and the drop-in center where we initially met the women, we were struck by how dissimilar the two facilities seemed. At the halfway house the women were nicely dressed and groomed, bustling around doing chores, attending meetings, and planning for a sober future in which they would live normative American middle-class lives. At the drop-in center most of the women carried their belongings in bags and backpacks; they looked homeless, many appeared to be high or otherwise intoxicated, and no one seemed to be working in a serious ways toward goals such as education or finding employment. Impressed by these differences, our initial plan was to carry out a comparative study of the two groups of women in order to understand why some pull their lives together while others remain stuck in homelessness, addiction, and misery. The problem with that plan, we soon found out, is that virtually all of the women we had met at one facility had been in the other facility at some point in the past—and often more than one point—and many of them moved on to the other facility over the course of the study's five years.

The five-year time frame allowed us unique opportunities to accompany women through cycles of ups and downs. We saw the same women sober and high, homeless and housed, employed and unemployed, in a supportive relationship and abused by a boyfriend, enthusiastically attending church and stigmatized by church members, involved on a daily basis with their children and out of those children's lives, sick and healthy, happy and despondent. Sometimes they told us how well things were going: perhaps they finally got housing or a kind boyfriend; stayed sober; had charges dropped; obtained health care, needed surgery, or better medication; qualified for food stamps; visited their children; landed a part-time job or a wonderful new caseworker; or reconciled with estranged family members. We have learned over the years that how well things are going one month or one year is unlikely to predict how things will go down the line. An individual sometimes looks and sounds like a poster child for the "working poor," the category used during the Clinton administration; that is, a worthy, hardworking, productive soul who with a bit of help will climb the rungs of America's economic ladder. But a year earlier or a year later, the same woman may look and sound and act strung out, down and out, "shit out of luck"—the unworthy, unproductive "welfare queen" or "crack whore" who cares more about dope than about getting a job or caring for her children. That these transitions are so commonplace suggests to us that the line between scraping by and not scraping by has become exceedingly porous in contemporary America.

Even when things seem to be going well, there are no happy endings in this community. After waiting years for a subsidized apartment, the housing Tonya moved into was infested with bedbugs. Joy, held up as a model of success when she graduated from the halfway house program, was back on the streets after her landlord took her rent check and then shut off the water and electricity on the same day that she was hit with food poisoning. Anasia landed a job as a home health aide—for a client who repeatedly called her by a racial slur. When Christine was laid off from her job after three years, she learned that her employer had not been paying into unemployment insurance. Daisy's purse was stolen the day she cashed her Social Security check. Vanessa's seemingly extraordinarily kind and solicitous boyfriend turned into a violent stalker who locked her in a room. Because Gloria's mail was stolen, she failed to receive and fill out a form to recertify her health care coverage. Francesca almost lost a foot to infection after an ostensibly minor surgery. Robin's daughter was raped while in foster care. The clinic assigned Elizabeth a new psychiatrist, who insisted on changing her medication—and the new medication made her so loopy that she fell asleep in the park and was sexually assaulted. And when Isabella called the police to protect her from a man who was trying to kick in her door, her identification check showed an outstanding warrant for failure to pay court fees and *she* was locked up.

We have come to understand that while many portals lead *into* lives of affliction, few lead out. The largest risk factor for sexual abuse is having been sexually abused in the past; the largest risk factor for poverty is already having been poor; the largest risk factor for incarceration is previous incarceration. Poverty and prison mark an individual both physically and legally. All the women we met have been turned away from housing because of their criminal records. Nearly all are toothless or nearly toothless in the wake of battering and malnutrition. Only four have been able to land steady jobs, and even these four earned less than a living wage. For too many Americans, a lifetime of abuse and affliction leads to an early death. Sadly, over 15 percent of the women released in 1995 from the Massachusetts state prison for women (MCI-Framingham) were dead by 2010; the average age at death was forty-four—more than thirty years younger than noncriminalized women of the same age cohort (Norton-Hawk, Sered, & Mastrorilli 2013).

THE CASTE OF THE ILL AND AFFLICTED

The women we describe in this book generally go unnoticed. Most do not sleep on the streets but are erratically housed, sometimes couch-surfing in the homes of friends and relatives, other times staying with a male acquaintance in exchange for sex, still other times renting a room or apartment until the rent money runs out. They do not look "criminal" or "crazy." They may serve your coffee at Dunkin Donuts, or they may be sitting next to you in the waiting area of the local emergency room. They represent the millions of Americans who are abused, sick, and in pain; are barely scraping by financially; are hooked on prescription or street drugs; and are likely to be drawn into a correctional system that takes away their freedom and their ability ever to obtain the types of employment that would allow them to achieve the American Dream. These women desperately want to live "happy" and "normal" lives; they want to raise their children, clean their houses, cook and bake, and be loved by a kind man who earns a legitimate salary. They want to "do the right thing." Most truly want "out" of a lifestyle that they know will eventually kill them, yet they remain trapped in the caste of the ill and afflicted.[2]

We use *caste* purposefully to get at the sense of finality: there is little chance of upward mobility for the women we met. As a consequence of the economic policies of the past several decades, increasing numbers of Americans have lost the middle- and working-class jobs that offered wages adequate for raising a family, benefits such as health insurance, some measure of job security, and the potential for advancement. Across the United States the gap between rich and poor has widened: smaller numbers of people are richer than ever, while growing numbers of people have seen their incomes decline. In vicious cycles, the effects of poverty are sustained across generations. The children of poor parents are substantially more likely than children of nonpoor parents to have a physical or mental disability that limits their activities (Kronstadt 2008), and having a child with chronic illnesses or disabilities is associated with greater poverty for parents (Batavia & Beaulaurier 2001).

As a term for describing certain types of social organization, *caste* emphasizes bodily classifications marked by recognizable external signs. Illness itself constitutes a physical marker. Rotten teeth (implying drug use), a chronic cough (implying smoking), obesity (implying lack of self-discipline), slurred speech (implying alcohol use), sexually transmitted infections (implying sexual deviance), odd behaviors such as talking to oneself (implying mental illness, a disease category that has long been stigmatized)—all of these signal caste in basic ways. Other castelike traits that we identify in this book include residential segregation ("ghettos"); concentration of lower-caste members in occupations dealing with dirt, sickness, or sex (one of the most common legal jobs held by the Boston women is that of a personal caregiver or nursing home assistant; one of the most common illegal jobs is sex work); and group affiliations such as legal status trumping individual characteristics and achievements. Race—an attribute perceived (erroneously) to be an immutable physical marker having to do not only with skin color but with personality traits and sexual behavior—is foundational to the American caste system. Even when African Americans become affluent, they are still "black" and subject to racial profiling (we return to matters of race in chapter 3).

We realize, of course, that not everyone who loses a job or is sexually assaulted ends up where Francesca ended up: miserable, sick, working in a strip club, and, eventually, in jail. In Francesca's case, the intersection of two powerful social forces—gender oppression and economic inequality—shaped her life trajectory. For Anasia and Gloria, two African American women, the intersection of racism with sexism and poverty practically guaranteed that they would join the caste of the ill and afflicted. While all women suffer from the effects of gender inequality, a woman who is sexually abused is more likely to become stuck in poverty if she lacks the resources to leave a bad marriage, move to a safer neighborhood, switch to another job, or elicit the support and sympathy of the police and judicial personnel. Following Kimberlé Crenshaw (1991) and work by other feminists of color, we recognize and appreciate the intersecting multiple identities that derive from social relations, history, and the operation of structures of power (Collins 2000, p. 18). Throughout this project we saw again and again that an individual can experience both oppression as a woman and privilege as a member of the professional class (as we the authors do); both privilege as white and oppression as poor (as Francesca did); both privilege as American-born and oppression as transgendered (as Ginger, whom we meet in chapter 4, did). At each juncture, individuals confront particular constellations of treatment and status, and develop particular perceptions and viewpoints regarding the world. Throughout this book we endeavor to expose—and to learn from—the advantages and disadvantages that result from various combinations of gender, sexual, health, race, class, and criminal status identities (Symington 2004).

PERSONAL FLAWS AND POOR CHOICES

Why do so many people continue to suffer so terribly in a country that boasts an extraordinarily sophisticated medical arsenal (indeed, the highest per capita medical spending in the world), extensive networks of mental health professionals and self-help therapeutic treatments, numerous child and social welfare agencies, high levels of church membership, government-funded faith-based programs, and the top incarceration rate on the planet (surely high enough to get the "bad guys" out of the way)? The women we describe in this book have spent years and, in some cases, decades moving in and out of homeless shelters, family shelters, drug courts, probation, parole, rehabilitation programs, mental health centers, detoxification facilities, emergency rooms, clinics, respite care, battered women's services, hospitals, welfare offices, WIC offices (for the USDA's Special Supplemental Nutrition Program for Women, Infants, and Children), Social Security (Supplemental Security Income [SSI] or Social Security Disability Insurance [SSDI]), psychiatric units, mental health centers, child welfare offices, family court, public housing, sober houses, substance abuse programs, faith-based agencies, prisons, and jails (Hopper et al. 1997). And yet, for the most part, the women do not escape membership in the caste of the ill and afflicted.

Following women through this institutional circuit, we have come to identify an extraordinarily broad cultural pattern—a spoken and unspoken social consensus—that attributes suffering to individual failings (cf. Sudbury 2005, p. xvi). Despite ostensibly different mandates (punishment, protection, helping, curing), the institutions on the circuit reinforce a cultural ethos in which pain and misery are considered products of idiosyncratic experience, personal flaws, and poor choices. Prisons, welfare offices, and clinics—albeit in different styles—promote the canon that individuals can choose their health, jobs, luck, and relationships—that we are responsible for our own misfortune.

While the actual life experiences of the women we have come to know are constrained by inflexible bureaucratic regimes, discriminatory policies, violent men, the international drug trade, and global economic forces, on the institutional circuit the message is that their suffering is the result of the choices that they personally make: the wrong men, wrong education, wrong drugs, wrong beliefs, and wrong relationships. Drilled in that message, the Boston women typically describe themselves as "needy": chronically ill; physically, emotionally, and genetically flawed; and as victims of specific men or particular, nasty caseworkers or parole officers—not as victims of gendered, racial, and economic inequalities that do not serve them well. We have rarely heard even the hint of a notion that misery is caused by the failure of the collective to address inequalities, poverty, environmental degradation, occupational hazards, stressful working conditions, and gendered violence, racism, sexism, or economic inequity;

by social structures or policies that create and reinforce inequality and animosities; or by the absence of a national commitment to human rights. To be clear—not all facilities and programs directly preach the message of personal responsibility for affliction. Rather, the totality of the institutional circuit's focus on the individual reinforces broader cultural notions that individuals are responsible for their own misery.

———————

The uncontested model of individual responsibility that is reiterated throughout the circuit (and indeed throughout the wider culture) not only fails to fix suffering caused by structural inequities, but actually leads to even greater distress when individuals feel that they, personally, have failed to achieve the American Dream. On the institutional circuit, women learn that their problems lie within themselves rather than outside in the real world, that their suffering is an expression of personal pathology rather than a manifestation of structural inequalities and violence. Within this ideological frame, an individual is understood to make bad choices because there is something wrong with her or with him. Bad choices made involuntarily because of physical, mental, or emotional flaws are treated medically. Bad choices made voluntarily, because of moral flaws, are treated with punishment. In line with that doctrine, the Boston women's misery is managed through mind-boggling amounts of drugs, therapy, Alcoholics Anonymous and Narcotics Anonymous meetings, and programs designed to boost women's self-esteem. When all of those fail, their misery often lands them in jail. It is not our intention to suggest that the women are without fault. They often make choices that, to us, seem to lead them ever deeper into lives of affliction. Rather, the doctrine of choice—as it is employed in American culture—presupposes that the individual is an autonomous social unit and that "good" choices are realistically available.

The institutional circuit is not, of course, a separate entity outside American culture. To the contrary, all of our major institutions rest upon and reinforce the American grand narrative of individualism (Albrecht 2012). Echoing the Protestant ethic, Americans have long been inclined to blame social problems on the individual's moral failures. With the ascent of modern medicine, those failures—while still carrying a moral valence—have increasingly come to be treated by doctors and pharmaceuticals. Medicalization— that is, characterizing problems or conditions in medical terms and adopting a medical approach to address those problems—resonates with long-standing

American values of individualism, experimentation, pragmatism, capitalism, and humanitarianism (Conrad & Schneider 1980; Crawford 2006). Susan Sontag is one of many observers of American society to argue that contemporary American culture embraces theories that assign to the sick individual responsibility for falling ill or not getting well (Sontag 2003). Although this discourse is most explicit in regard to HIV/AIDS, the court of public opinion often blames illness on "poor lifestyle choices," and the sick (especially the chronically ill and those suffering from invisible illnesses such as diabetes or mental illness) are likely to be blamed for neglecting to take care of themselves, failing to comply with doctor's orders, or perhaps faking illness in order to get government assistance (Hay 2010). A good fit for conservative economic policies whose proponents are looking to cut government spending on social services, this model absolves government and corporate leadership of responsibility for instituting and enforcing environmental regulations that foster public health, and it underpins the War on Drugs, a "war" aimed at individual drug users rather than at the underlying social causes of the drug epidemic.

We have come to understand that medicalization and criminalization are two sides of the same coin, namely, the definition and management of suffering as manifestations of personal flaws. Both medicalization and criminalization rest on an ideology of personal responsibility that obscures the structural causes of suffering. Processes of labeling and treating certain people or actions as criminal change over time and are produced within relations of social dominance. Behaviors that are acceptable or even valorous in some cultures are criminalized in others. In the contemporary United States both medicalization and criminalization have proven to be greedy social forces that continuously expand the attributes and phenomena swept into their nets. Sadness and anger, menstruation and menopause, pregnancy and lactation, passivity and aggression, being too thin or too fat, consuming alcohol or junk food, working too much or not enough, assaulting others or being assaulted have all become targets of pharmaceutical interventions, both legal and illicit (Conrad 1992). At the same time, we have expanded our ideas regarding criminality to the point that we lock up a larger percentage of our population than we have in any previous era, with drug-related charges heavily driving that increase.

CAPTIVES OF THE INSTITUTIONAL CIRCUIT

We coin the term *institutional captives* to describe people entrapped in the institutional circuit. While all Americans come into contact with various public and private institutions, homeless people are more likely to use mental health services and emergency rooms; Americans who have received welfare are more likely to be drawn into the correctional system; and participation in drug rehabilitation programs is linked to higher likelihood of involvement with child welfare offices. Institutional captives experience the penal-welfare-medical system as one interlocking metasystem ("the system") having enormous practical and ideological power.

Not all institutional captives are treated in the same way. Quite the contrary, the same social inequalities that poor and abused Americans encounter in their homes, communities, and streets are replicated on the institutional circuit when formal and informal policies reinforce racial, gender, and class polarization and conflict. Welfare recipients—the very poorest Americans—are treated with more suspicion than, for instance, recipients of retirement benefits (Social Security and Medicare) or veterans' benefits (cf. Reiman 2010). African Americans and Hispanic Americans are more likely than white Americans to be arrested and incarcerated, a situation that Michelle Alexander has described as "the new Jim Crow." Within prisons and homeless shelters rigid gender segregation is the largely unquestioned norm, highly gendered standards for appropriate behavior are enforced (cf. Britton 2003) and LGBTQ people suffer additional layers of discrimination, harassment, and pain. Throughout the circuit, the people at the very top institutional levels—where policies are set—are likely to be white, male, and affluent, while those at the bottom of institutional hierarchies employed in jobs that engage most directly with institutional captives in jails, nursing homes, and rehab facilities tend to be low-income men and women of color (Britton 2003).

We have struggled with the language we use to describe the women we have come to know. Our nomenclature dilemma is not new. In their classic 1934 study of women released from the same Massachusetts prison in which most of the women of our project also were incarcerated, Sheldon Glueck and Eleanor Touroff Glueck (1934) rejected the label "criminals," arguing that very few of the women had actually committed a significant crime. Much like women confined in jails and prisons today, most were locked up for acts of social deviance such as running away from home or prostitution. The Gluecks offered the term *les misérables* as a way of emphasizing that poverty and problematic family situations were more salient than the petty crimes for which women tended to be locked up. We searched for an English translation of les misérables but could not identify a word that expresses comparable complexities of personal wretchedness and subordinate social and economic status. From the start we eliminated offender (women are far more likely to suffer offense than to commit offenses). Victim carries the stigma of passivity in a culture that values action, draws attention to the recipient of violence rather than the perpetrator, and discounts the many ways in which women actively defend themselves and their children. Homeless is inaccurate; although most of the women are insecurely housed, few sleep on the streets. Elizabeth, whom we introduce in chapter 2, is adamant that she is not a homeless person ("being homeless is not who I am"); rather, because of circumstances, she has "been in the homeless life for ten years." When we asked several project participants what they call women in their situation, several offered losers or fucked up. We rejected the first as erasing the enormous victories involved in staying alive; the latter we rejected because it reflects the same blame-the-individual outlook that led us to reject victim.

In light of the significance of sexual abuse in their lives as well as the pervasive gender segregation that is taken for granted on the institutional circuit, we decided to go simply with "women," adding modifying words such as in "Boston women" or "the women we met during this project" for clarity.

CANARIES IN THE COAL MINE

The women we describe in this book are canaries in the coal mine of contemporary American society in that they represent the vanguard of the caste of the ill and afflicted. Early in life they entered the spiral of poor jobs and poor health, and they became stuck, despite—and in some cases because of—institutional interventions. Many Americans who become ill, or who are assaulted or lose their jobs, turn to social service agencies for short-term assistance with a discrete problem, receive useful assistance, and move on with their lives. Those of us fortunate enough to have marketable job skills, college degrees, supportive families, and strong social networks are less likely to become stuck. Still, while we Americans like to believe in the power of the individual to take control of his (sic) life, the fact is that nearly anyone who experiences a sufficient amount of bad luck over a sufficiently long time is a candidate for the caste of the ill and afflicted.

We have written this book because of our concern that more and more Americans are becoming actual or potential caste members. Indeed, during the years of this project we witnessed the lines for free lunches lengthen at the women's drop-in center, and we saw more and more people waiting in those lines who have jobs but are still not able to scrape by. According to the Current Population Survey (DeNavas-Walt, Proctor, & Smith 2013), 15 percent of Americans—or roughly 46.5 million people, including more than 16 million children—live at or below the government-defined poverty line ($23,492 for a family of four). Double or triple that number live marginally above the poverty line, not earning sufficient funds to make ends meet. Between 2009 and 2011, the wealthiest 7 percent of Americans became wealthier by 28 percent, while the rest of the country became poorer by 4 percent (Fry & Taylor 2013). An estimated 21 million Americans are classified as abusing or being dependent on psychotropic substances (SAMHSA 2012). One out of every fifteen young adults has been diagnosed as seriously mentally ill (U.S. Government Accountability Office 2008).[3] An estimated one-third of all American women have been subjected to sexual or physical abuse (Friedan, Degutis, & Spivak 2010). And, *both nationally and internationally, greater economic inequality, regardless of the absolute wealth or poverty of the society overall, correlates with more homicides, mental illness, illegal drug use, and incarceration* (Wilkinson & Pickett 2009).

———

The Boston women are canaries in the coal mine in a second sense. In comparison to other U.S. states, Massachusetts has comparatively low rates of incarceration and high rates of health care access and coverage. Women (and men) in Texas, California, and indeed most other states are likely to receive less health care and more punishment than Massachusetts women. As we are writing this book, much of the country seems poised to move in the direction Massachusetts has taken. The National Patient Protection and Affordable Care Act of 2010 ("Obamacare") is modeled on Massachusetts's health care insurance reform law of 2006. And, after far too many years of rising prison population, there are signs that America's race to incarcerate may be slowing down. Attorney General Eric Holder has called for scaling back sentences for drug-related crimes. Due to prison overcrowding, California, the state with the largest number of people behind bars, has been ordered by a panel of federal judges to reduce the its prison population by approximately 10,000.

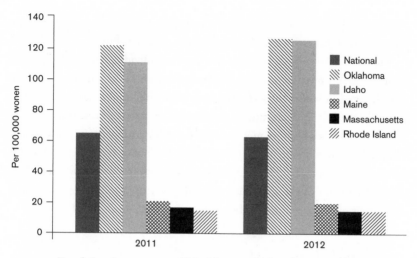

FIGURE 1. Female imprisonment rates, United States and selected states, 2011–2012. Oklahoma and Idaho have the highest female imprisonment rate (per 100,000 women) in the country, while Rhode Island and Massachusetts have the lowest. *Source:* Bureau of Justice Statistics 2013.

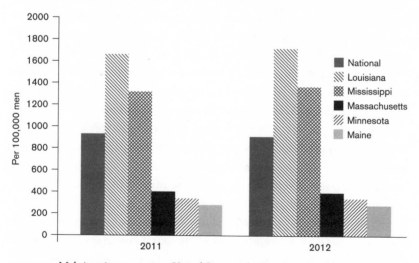

FIGURE 2. Male imprisonment rates, United States and selected states, 2011–2012. Louisiana and Mississippi have the highest male imprisonment rate (per 100,000 men) in the country, while Maine and Minnesota have the lowest. *Source:* Bureau of Justice Statistics 2013.

And the White House has outlined a new drug policy that shifts the focus from criminal justice to health care responses to drug abuse.

Medical interventions aimed at treating the individual are certainly more benign than criminalization that is intended to punish the individual. But we have learned in Massachusetts that even with the best of intentions—and virtually all of the doctors, nurses, social workers, caseworkers, and even correctional officers whom we met are indeed well intentioned—individualized treatment cannot cure structural inequalities. In the words of a Massachusetts primary care doctor who has worked with drug addicts for many years, "We are all cognizant of the social determinants of illness and made aware on a daily basis of our very limited ability to do anything meaningful about it."

OVERVIEW OF THE BOOK

We have arranged the chapters in a loosely chronological order following the typical sequence in which the women tended to encounter or recognize particular problems and particular institutions. This is not a linear trajectory; the social forces that set the women on the path of misery do not go away once they are medicated, in therapy, or locked up. Chapter 1 picks up Francesca's story of gender inequalities and sexual violence. In chapter 2 we look at poverty and homelessness through the lens of Elizabeth's experiences on the institutional circuit. Chapter 3 tells the story of Anasia's encounters with residential segregation and racist attitudes and dictates.

The second half of the book addresses the dominant ideologies and practices used to explain and manage suffering in the contemporary United States. Chapter 4 explores the path to and consequences of Ginger's licit and illicit drug use in the wider context of medicalization. In Chapter 5 we introduce Gloria and argue that the popular therapeutic language of victimization, trauma, and PTSD (posttraumatic stress disorder) diverts attention from the structural causes of suffering, emphasizing instead the personal flaws of unfortunate individuals. In chapter 6 we follow Joy in and out of drug rehab programs. Through Joy's travels, we show how the core ideology of the institutional circuit is made explicit in the ubiquitous Twelve Step programs that preach the doctrine of individual responsibility for one's failings and the message that happiness and healing can come only through turning oneself over to a higher power. Chapter 7 focuses on Kahtia and her children and argues that social inequalities and poorly conceived institutional interventions perpetuate membership in the caste of the ill and afflicted through to the next generation. Finally, in chapter 8, we visit Isabella in prison and look more closely at prisons as the anchor of the institutional circuit and the ultimate setting for the criminalization of affliction.

We conclude the book with a human rights framework for moving forward. The appendix presents further details about the project and the project women.

CHAPTER I

"Joey Spit on Me"

How Gender Inequality and Sexual Violence Make Women Sick

We have an abundance of rape and violence against women in this country and on this Earth, though it's almost never treated as a civil rights or human rights issue, or a crisis, or even a pattern.

—Rebecca Solnit, "The Longest War Is the One against Women" (2013)

Men—they don't want to leave me . . . they want to control me.

—Robin

Francesca's father came to the United States to live the American dream. An Italian sailor, he jumped ship and swam to shore in Massachusetts, where he married a woman from a well-established Italian American family. Francesca describes her father as "a typical macho Italian man." From the outside, they were a stable and successful blue-collar family. Her parents owned their home; Dad worked at the same job his entire adult life, and Mom stayed home with the children. Francesca's early memories are of festivals at the local church, her mother's traditional recipes for Easter lamb and Italian meatballs, and her father's stories from the Italian American social club. But below the surface her family was sliding into a spiral of illness and affliction. From as early as Francesca can remember, her mother was sick: throat cancer, eye disease, and congestive heart failure, trips to the psychiatric hospital and suicide attempts. It was up to Francesca, as the only daughter still living at home, to clean up the blood and bandage her mother's slit wrists.

By the time Francesca was thirteen, things were going very wrong. Her "scumbag" older brother began molesting her. Her parents learned of the sexual abuse from the pediatrician who discovered anal warts (a symptom of human papillomavirus [HPV] infection). In response to the abuse, Francesca was put on psychiatric medication; her brother was not held to account for his behavior. Thirty years later Francesca still shakes when recalling how her parents instructed her to tell Child Welfare Services that it was her late grandfather—not her brother—who had molested her. Before her fourteenth birthday she ran away from home to escape the abuse. By the age of fifteen she had met an older man, and as soon as she turned eighteen, she married him. Together they had two sons; a third pregnancy was aborted at her husband's insistence. Francesca recalls the years when the boys were young as the happiest in her life. She loved, and still loves, being a mother.

For ten years or so Francesca supported the family, working as a waitress while her husband used the family funds to support his drug habit. A violent man, he beat her up badly and often, kicking out her teeth, breaking her ribs, and stabbing her in the stomach, causing her to undergo a hysterectomy. Just as bad, according to Francesca, he "destroyed my self-esteem," repeatedly telling her that she was fat and that no other man would ever want her. Despite it all, Francesca managed to work at a series of low-paying, physically strenuous jobs through her late twenties. When her father became terminally ill with cancer, she quit her job to nurse him. At his death, he left the family home to her to live in, and pay the mortgage on. Several years later, "out of the blue someone from the bank showed up," and she and her children were told that they had to move out immediately. It turned out that her husband had fed his drug habit with the money she had given him to pay the mortgage.

By the time Francesca's marriage ended, she was living with multiple, painful chronic conditions, some the direct legacy of her husband's violence: osteoarthritis (a consequence of his beatings), degenerative disk disease with chronic pain and swelling in her back, a broken nose that interfered with her sleep, broken teeth, and panic attacks. She also was diagnosed with hepatitis C and rheumatoid arthritis.[1] Although the hepatitis C is destroying her liver, Francesca is more worried about the visible conditions, especially the rotten teeth and the scarred skin that make it difficult for her to find a job or, in her words, a "good man." Doctors prescribed Percocet for the chronic pain that she developed from the beatings, as well as a pharmacopeia of psychotropic drugs for "my anxiety and bi-polar." It did not take long for her use of Percocet and anti-anxiety medication to escalate into addiction. When the doctors wouldn't write any more prescriptions, she turned to the streets for her Percocet.

In 2001 Francesca served her first prison sentence for larceny. While she certainly was willing to shoplift or sell an occasional prescription pill in order to scrape by, this charge was tied to her husband having passed bad checks in her name. During the year in jail, her brother (the same one who had molested Francesca) requested and received custody of her children. The state paid him $1,000 a month for each child, and to this day Francesca believes that he wanted the children only for the money. Upon leaving prison, she found that she had lost her Section VIII (federally subsidized) housing eligibility. For the next ten years Francesca cycled in and out of jail, shelters, temporary housing, lousy relationships, and jobs like the strip club gig that ended in misery.

CYCLES OF VIOLENCE

When Francesca first told us about her life, we couldn't understand why she left an abusive father and brother only to marry an abusive husband. Nearly all of the women in the project have suffered multiple sexual assaults. With very few exceptions they spent their childhood years in households where male violence against girls and women was commonplace. Nearly all witnessed fathers, step-fathers, or mother's boyfriends physically hurt and psychologically humiliate and control their mothers. Almost all have been raped as adults or been involved in relationships with battering men, or both.

In their encounters with gendered violence the Boston women are not unique. According to the 2010 National Intimate Partner and Sexual Violence Survey (Black et al. 2011), in the United States, on average, 24 people per minute are victims of rape, physical violence, or stalking by an intimate partner; more than 1 million women are raped yearly. Nearly 1 in 5 women has been raped at some time in her life; 1 in 4 women has been a victim of severe physical violence by an intimate partner in her lifetime; 1 in 6 women has experienced stalking victimization during her lifetime; and almost 70 percent of female victims experienced some form of intimate partner violence for the first time before the age of twenty-five (Black et al. 2011). Across the United States an estimated 30 percent of women have been targets of sexual or physical abuse, and nearly 1 in 5 girls ages fourteen to seventeen has been the victim of a sexual assault or attempted sexual assault. A history of sexual assault increases the likelihood of further sexual assault (Finkelhor et al. 2009).

———

Sexual assault is not simply a deviant act by a deviant man against an exceptionally unfortunate woman. Rather, it is part of a social cycle in which systemic gender inequality produces gendered violence that then reinforces gender inequality.

Gendered violence is always embedded in wider landscapes of inequality. Examining a wide range of cultures around the world, anthropologist Peggy Sanday (2003) found that the incidence of rape is lower in societies in which men are raised in peaceful, stable environments with an ethos of mutual respect and cooperation between men and women. Conversely, societies that promote gender inequality have more cases of domestic abuse and violence overall (Tracy 2007). Turning to the United States, we observe that American women have the same responsibilities of citizenship as men do (women and men are held to the same set of laws and pay the same taxes), yet women earn 77 cents on each dollar earned by men (White House Council on Women and Girls 2012). For American women, the power to make their own reproductive decisions is limited and in some cases outright denied. While American women have made strides in the public sphere, they remain grossly underrepresented in the highest levels of government where the most consequential decisions are made. The United States currently ranks 81st among nations worldwide in the inclusion of women in government, and 22nd in the economic, political, health, and education status of women (Hausmann, Tyson, & Zahidi 2012).

Gendered violence begets more gendered violence. For the perpetrator, carrying out an act of aggression with impunity feeds a sense of entitlement or, at the very least, a sense that one can get away with it. The majority of rapists and batterers are serial offenders who abuse more than one woman over their lives (Tracy 2007). Donna, a high-energy white woman in her forties, grew up in a home in which her father and brothers were physically and sexually abusive to her and her sister. "My mother was too afraid to say anything," she told us. "My mother would send one of the girls into the bathroom with toilet paper for my father. We all knew what was going on." Although she left home to escape her father's abuse, she quickly found herself married to a controlling and violent man. Donna explains, "I think the reason he hits me is because his father always hit his mom." Together with other structures of dominance, rape is a forceful weapon in the wider arsenal of tools used to generate and preserve gender inequality (Brownmiller 1975; see also A. Davis 1981, esp. p. 178; Hunnicutt 2009). As a "cultural mechanism for inducing a significant transformation of consciousness" (Morris 1991, p. 181), rape reinforces gender stereotypes of masculinity and of femininity.

As one might expect in light of Francesca's childhood experiences, battering fathers tend to be authoritarian, controlling, self-centered, and undermining of the mothers. They are also many times more likely than nonbatterers to sexually abuse their children, especially their daughters (Bancroft, Silverman, & Ritchie 2012). Thus Francesca's "typical macho Italian father" ruled over her timid, ill, and eventually suicidal mother at the same time that her "scumbag" older brother was raping her. Like many abused girls, Francesca criticizes her mother rather than her father for allowing the abuse to happen. Although it sounds to us as if her father held all of the power in the house, Francesca has elevated him to the realm of sainthood—especially now that he is dead. In blaming her mother more than her father, Francesca follows the public tendency to hold mothers more responsible than fathers for protecting their children from a cruel world over which parents have little real control. Still today, when Francesca considers the misery in her life and the lack of adequate assistance with money, housing, and personal safety, she, like most of the other project women, tends to blame (female) caseworkers, nurses, and parole officers far more than she blames the (male) politicians and power brokers who actually make the policies and control the national purse strings.

The physical and psychic scars of sexual violence direct the attention of the women who bear them to their gender, setting them up for lives in which they are never simply "human" but always "woman," an identity largely defined in terms of sexual victimization and gynecological suffering. What we are describing here is *gender overdetermination*: a social process in which cultural categories of gender supersede individual experience and identity (Boddy 1988; Sered and Norton-Hawk 2013). Gender overdetermination intersects in complex ways with other statuses and identities. In a multi-city study, Stephanie Riger and Margaret Gordon (2010) found that women with the fewest resources— the elderly, members of ethnic minorities, and those with low incomes— carry the heaviest burden of fear of victimization and a heightened sense of powerlessness. While for some women, abuse and its aftermath can lead to new kinds of resilience or to meaningful advocacy and activism, few of the women we have come to know see possibilities for jobs, happiness, or self-fulfillment that are not constrained by gender. Their gendered pain becomes the veil through which they experience their own bodies and lives.

Sexual abuse has broad and long-term consequences that function to perpetuate social inequalities. Childhood abuse is correlated with bruises, fractures, urinary tract infections, delayed physical growth, neurological damage, chronic fatigue, altered immune function, hypertension, obesity, depression, suicidal thoughts and attempts, risky behaviors, substance abuse, and in extreme cases, death (Herrera & McCloskey 2001; White, Koss, & Kazdin 2011). Women who have been abused by intimate partners or who have been sexually assaulted are more likely than other women to suffer from chronic pelvic pain, fertility problems, high rates of pregnancy complications and perinatal death, gastrointestinal disorders, arthritis, invasive cervical cancer, hypertension, urinary tract infections, anxiety, and sexually transmitted infections (Martin, Macy, & Young 2011).

A history of having been abused is correlated with a lifetime of earning less money, missing more days of work, and a greater likelihood of becoming homeless (Dáil 2012, p. 17). A 23-city report by the U.S. Conference of Mayors (2007) confirmed that domestic violence is the primary cause of homelessness for women. For Francesca, poor health clearly renders her unemployable, which makes her more dependent on men and thus more vulnerable to additional sexual violence. For Francesca, as for many women, the physical and emotional suffering resulting from rape, abuse, and sexual coercion led to use of drugs and alcohol. Women who have been raped or abused are more likely than other women to use licit and illicit drugs, to be charged with a crime, and to be incarcerated (McDaniels-Wilson & Belknap 2008; Pelissier & Jones 2006). The impact of violence is cumulative: women who have experienced or witnessed greater numbers of abusive events report higher rates of eating-related problems, greater incidence of STDs and hepatitis, overall poorer self-rated health status, earlier involvement in crime, and more arrests. In this way, violence thrusts women into the caste of the ill and afflicted.

Criminalized women are twice as likely as other American women to report childhood sexual abuse (45% versus 24%) and more than three times more likely to report family violence while growing up (48% versus 14%) (Messina & Grella 2006). Like Francesca, nearly all criminalized women have experienced poverty, abuse, insecure housing, chronic physical and mental distress, separation from their children, and a host of day-to-day degradations and misfortunes. Nationally, at least 70 percent of incarcerated women report having been raped at some point in their lives, typically more than once and often by multiple abusers; more than 10 percent report gang rape; and 22 percent report anal rape (McDaniels-Wilson & Belknap 2008).

As Francesca learned from her first experience with the institutional circuit, the dominant model for explaining these connections singles out childhood abuse as causing lasting psychological damage that in turn leads to drug use and further victimization. While this causal chain fits the American narrative of individual responsibility for suffering, connections between gender violence and incarceration are far more structural. Running away from home in the wake of sexual abuse launches girls into environments permeated with gendered violence, both on the street and in juvenile facilities. Children who suffer sexual assault are less likely to succeed in school, less likely ever to earn a living wage, and more likely to be incarcerated (Child Welfare Information Services 2008). In fact, running away from home—often to escape abuse in households dominated by violent men—is the charge in the first arrest for nearly a quarter of girls in the juvenile justice system. According to Meda Chesney-Lind and Lisa Pasko (2004, p. 28), "Young women, a large number of whom are on the run from sexual abuse and parental neglect, are forced by the very statutes designed to protect them [statutes disallowing juveniles from leaving custodial parents] into the lives of escaped convicts. Unable to enroll in school or take a job to support themselves because they fear detection [which may result in their being returned to the abusive household], young female runaways often turn to or are forced onto the streets. Here they engage in panhandling, petty theft, and occasional prostitution to survive." On the streets, women are vulnerable to harassment, violence, exploitation, and drug use, all of which drag them into the correctional circuit, where, far too frequently, they experience further abuse.

Girls and women who have experienced abuse are also more likely to be drawn into prostitution (Martin, Hearst, & Widome 2010). Estimates suggest that among women working in prostitution, as many as 75 percent were sexually abused as girls (Nixon et al. 2002). In Francesca's case, the constellation of aborted education, meager employment prospects, emotional exhaustion, and immersion in a cultural setting in which sex has more to do with power than with love set her up for sex work. And while paid sex work is not infrequently portrayed as romantic (think of the film *Pretty Woman*), lucrative (though this is true only in the rare cases of famous madams who supply prostitutes to politicians and celebrities), empowering (think *Breakfast at Tiffany's*), or funny (as in, for example, *Deuce Bigalow: Male Gigolo*), in our many conversations and interactions with women who have worked in prostitution, we have never glimpsed a hint of romance, humor, resistance against social norms, big bucks, or pride. The women we know make it clear that sex is not in any way equivalent to other paid or unpaid labor; to work in prostitution, a prostitute must disengage the self or "go numb." While "viccing" (cheating or victimizing) male customers sometimes may be seen as a form of resistance against male power: "Ironically, it is this very resistance which serves to (re) produce them as 'criminal' women at risk for violent retaliation" (Maher 2000, p. 130). The death rate among women in prostitution has been estimated at forty times higher than that of the general population, and a mortality survey of more than 1,600 women in prostitution found that no other population of American women has a death rate even approaching that of prostitutes (Farley 2004).

FRANCESCA

After the strip club gig ended, Francesca picked up a series of day jobs giving out free samples of juice "from an Amazonian rainforest fruit known since the dawn of time for its rejuvenating properties," selling beauty supplies from a table outside a tourist information center, and loading the truck for a one-man moving company run by a Christian pastor she dated for a few months. Homeless, Francesca couldn't provide a place to live for her kids (one in his late teens, the other in his early twenties), but she did her level best to help them network with potential employers and to arrange for them to stay with friends and pay for their cell phones so that they could stay in touch with her. When her younger son was arrested for assault and battery (with a great deal of pride she told us that he had beaten up a man who was trying to hurt a girl), she met him at the police station and put money in his canteen so that he could buy coffee and snacks in jail.

Within a year she met Chris. His blond hair, blue eyes, and wiry build made it easy for Francesca to fall in love with him. In a whirlwind of dress shopping and flower arranging, she married him in a small ceremony on the beach followed by a party at a local karaoke bar. In the first months of their life together, she was delighted with what seemed a Christmas-card home life: he lived with his extended family in a small town two hours away from the drugs and temptations of Boston. Francesca moved in, hoping that her children would join the household and that they could live like "a real family" again.

But things soon turned sour. Because their house was not within walking distance from any town, Francesca depended on Chris's family for rides to the store, to work, or to Boston to see her children. Chris wanted to be with her "every minute," carrying on if she went out without him for even a few minutes. As things deteriorated, Chris began insulting her, pushing her buttons by calling her "fat ass" and "ugly," and accusing her of cheating on him. One morning he broke her cell phone and removed the chip (SIM card) with her phone numbers, making it nearly impossible for her to call on friends for help in finding another place to live. Hitchhiking and begging rides, she returned to Boston and moved in with an acquaintance. That arrangement seemed to be working out until Chris called the police with a "tip" that there were drugs in that apartment. There were no drugs, but the police checked everyone's identification, and Francesca was locked up on an outstanding warrant—she had not been able to pay restitution on a breaking-and-entering conviction ten years earlier. While she was in prison, the friend she had been staying with was evicted, and all of Francesca's possessions, including her ID and her dentures, were thrown out.

After serving a brief jail sentence she tried to look for a job, but with no teeth or decent clothes she was unemployable. Out of desperation she reunited with Chris, who by that time had moved out of his family's house. The two stayed for a few days at a time with various relatives and then settled in for several weeks with her younger son's friend. That worked reasonably well until Chris tried to knock down the door of a neighbor. As had become our routine, Francesca called us and asked us to pick her up. With all of her earthly possessions in one small plastic bag, she next stayed for a few days each at the homes of various friends, moving on when Chris stalked and found her. During this time she contracted pneumonia and her hepatitis C began to flare up. Her stomach became visibly distended; she had pain in her side and several episodes of vomiting. By early winter her feet and legs had swollen up, and she was making frequent trips to her doctor and the hospital. At one visit she was told that she might have a blood clot in her heart, and an appointment was scheduled for her to see a cardiologist two weeks later. Francesca's posture changed—she no longer stood up straight. Even her hair lost its luster. With none of the bravado she had displayed when we first met her, Francesca sighed, "I'm just tired of everything."

―――――――

Frequent trips to doctors and hospitals became routine for Francesca. Her need for medical treatment was driven both by the violence and poverty in her life and by her sense that she needed a doctor's validation in order to receive recognition as well as medication for her pain. Over the next few months Francesca lost close to thirty pounds, her stomach became bloated, and she developed rectal bleeding. The doctor told her that she had "a mass the size of a small apple and probably colon cancer," and scheduled her for a colonoscopy. The afternoon of the colonoscopy Francesca called us from the hospital in a panic. She had spent the previous night trying to sleep on an air mattress on the floor of her son's girlfriend's parents' apartment, where she had carried out her colonoscopy preparation according to the instructions she received (instructions that did not take into account that she would be sharing a bathroom with six other adults and a baby). The apartment was located a good thirty minutes by car and ninety minutes by public transportation from the Boston hospital, so she had arranged with a friend of her son (one of the only people she knew who had a car) to drive her to and from the appointment. However, when it was time for her to be picked up at the hospital, he didn't show, and the hospital would not allow her to leave without an adult escort (which is the typical protocol for procedures that involve sedation). "Please," she asked us, "could you come pick me up?"

Knowing firsthand how miserable the whole colonoscopy experience is even in the best of circumstances, we drove posthaste to the hospital, where a forlorn Francesca was sitting on a bench waiting for us to pick her up and walk with her to her primary care doctor's office in another wing of the hospital complex. Earlier in the day she had spoken to a nurse in his office and had arranged for her doctor to leave a prescription for Percocet at the desk. The envelope with her name on it, however, contained only a form for blood tests, and no prescriptions for pain medication. We sat, and sat, and sat while the receptionist looked around the office for the prescription. After an hour during which Francesca looked as if she would melt in her chair (she had not yet eaten that day), the nurse came out and called us into an examining room. Francesca explained what had happened, the nurse went out to speak to the doctor, and after another hour of waiting, the doctor came in, barely glanced at Francesca, and told her that he was not comfortable giving her Percocet, that she should take 800 milligrams of Motrin instead. Half in tears with postcolonoscopy exhaustion, she reminded him that when she was in his office the week before, she had told him that she had been taking Motrin for her arthritis and that he had told her to stop because she had taken far too much. Barely listening to her recounting (his attention was on the computer screen), he wrote a prescription for Motrin and told her she would need to go to the pain clinic. He left the room, and we sat and waited for another half hour, thinking he would return with a referral. Deflated, Francesca (more sensible than I) realized he would not be coming back; the medical assistant soon confirmed that "he was finished" with us. Not only did Francesca not receive a referral that day, but six months later the doctor still had not met with her to go over the colonoscopy results. We still do not know why.

At the time, about two years into our project, we could not comprehend what happened at the doctor's office. In retrospect, we understand that the doctor assumed that Francesca was "pill-seeking." Though young, the doctor must have known that by turning her away, there were two possible outcomes: she'd go to an emergency room (at great cost to the health care system), or she'd buy pain pills illegally on the street, putting herself into the dangerous hands of drug dealers and setting herself up for another prison sentence.

———

Francesca prides herself on being a "survivor." Finished with Chris, she moved in with a friend whom she had met in prison. Known as "Mama Fran" to the women of MCI-Framingham, Francesca embraced the opportunity to help out a former associate who was suffering from debilitating depression. In return for a place to stay, Francesca took over care of her friend's household and children. Francesca's younger son, now twenty and the father of an infant, moved in with them as well. Delighted to be a grandmother, Francesca regained much of her old bravado, revamped her wardrobe, and cut down on her Percocet use during her grandchild's visits.

In the summer of 2011 she met Joey, and Francesca's old exuberant persona returned in full force. "Joey is the love of my life!" she gushed. "He knows how to treat women. He buys me things and kisses me on the forehead and tells me that I am beautiful and deserve good things." A short, bald ex-con who had been out of prison for almost three years, Joey had a steady job and lived in a two-bedroom apartment furnished with an air mattress, an enormous television, and little else. Within a month of their meeting she moved in with him. Joey was generous to Francesca's children, warmly welcoming them for weekend visits. In Francesca's words, Joey was "a family man," and from the start she looked forward to celebrating a "real Christmas"—her first in a long time—with "my man and my kids."

High on the list of Joey's good qualities was his promise to support her so that she could take care of her health problems. Within a few months of meeting Joey, she planned to have surgery to fix her teeth, nose, throat, back, and hip (all injuries caused by her ex-husband). Before she could get to these surgeries, however, she had to take care of an immediately pressing health issue: flying debris during a storm scratched her cornea. Once her eye healed, she had surgery to remove all of her teeth and grind down and fix the bones in her upper mouth.

Christmas 2011 was a big day for Francesca. The living room—still empty of furniture—had plenty of room for the elaborately decorated tree and the piles of Christmas gifts Francesca had obtained through a local charity. We arrived just in time to see her son charge into the living room to peer inside his Christmas stocking (Francesca had filled it with candy and cigarettes). Beaming with pride, Francesca unwrapped the Chanukah cookies she had bought especially for Susan. Her e-mail message on Christmas proclaimed: "♥ IM TRULY BLESSED AND I GET TO SPEND TIME WITH BOTH MY KIDS TONIGHT AND MY MAN. . . . FAMILY IS [WHERE] ITS @. . . . CANT PUT A PRICE TAG ON THAT . . . (PRICELESS) ♥"

Like nearly all of the other Boston women, Francesca craves a life that matches her idealized vision of middle-class gender normativity. When she and her friends speculate about what their lives will be like in five years or ten years, they offer one of only two scenarios: either things will stay as bad as they are now and they likely will be dead; or they will live with their children in a *Leave It to Beaver*–style, 1950s house with a white picket fence and a friendly family pet. Francesca on occasion allows herself to dream aloud: "I will own a house, have a dog and my two boys with me." As both of her boys became fathers over the study's five years, her dream home evolved to include cooking and baking for her grandchildren when they come for frequent and lengthy sleepovers.

Once her mouth, eye, and various other body parts healed, Francesca felt healthier than she had in a long time. She worked for a while at a diner owned by an Italian family. Thrilled to be serving up authentic Italian food, Francesca treated us to a platter of spaghetti and sauce. But the job was very part-time with no real schedule: the boss would call her in only when the restaurant needed her, and she was paid under the table. When that job petered out, she was hired at a Dunkin Donuts where she worked erratic, long shifts at the whim of the manager. Standing at work exacerbated bone spurs in her foot. Her doctor gave her an orthopedic boot to wear, but the boot caused her to trip at work. She was not called back in. Without a job she was dependent on Joey for food, shelter, and pocket money. While he sometimes spontaneously gave her twenty dollars for a "mani-pedi" (Francesca loves bright patterned nails), at other times he would "call me a fat cunt" or "say my cooking is bad and throw it out the window" and "throw it [the new pocketbook, manicure, shoes, etc.] back in my face." On one occasion, "Joey spit on me. He doesn't trust women."

Living with Joey did allow her to arrange surgery for her foot. But in late April 2012, when Joey kicked her out and we came to pick her up, she was standing on the curb with her possessions in a few bags and her foot still in a cast. After a few half-hearted declarations of "Joey doesn't deserve a woman like me," Francesca fell into an uncharacteristic silence. Per doctor's orders, she kept her foot elevated—propped up on the dashboard of the car as we drove her back to the apartment of the friend she had been staying with before she moved in with Joey.

VICTIMS, PERPETRATORS, AND THE SOCIAL FOUNDATIONS OF SEXUAL VIOLENCE

Why—despite our society's efforts to help victims of violence—do Francesca and so many other women continue to suffer assaults, abuse, sexual exploitation, and rape? The federal Violence Against Women Act, signed into law by President Bill Clinton on September 13, 1994, increased penalties for repeat sex offenders, trained law enforcement officers to deal with victims of sexual offenses, and established the National Domestic Violence Hotline. Most cities like Boston have police, social workers, psychologists, battered women's shelters, rape crisis hotlines, mandatory reporting requirements—surely these have solved the problem of violence against women. Yet notwithstanding public proclamations that raise awareness of childhood sexual abuse, date rape, and domestic battering, mainstream social responses to sexual violence have not been particularly helpful; they have not changed the culture of violence that endangers women, children, and many men; and rates of gender violence have not declined.

Despite strong evidence linking gender inequality to higher levels of violence, contemporary American law and culture continue to address gender violence as an individual tragedy rather than a product of inequalities or structural violence. During the years Francesca lived with her ex-husband, she was a "frequent flyer" at her local emergency room. "They [the hospital staff] knew what was going on," she told us. Often, they would admit her for a day or two "to give me a break." For the most part, the staff treated her well, but hospitals do not have the resources to provide financial independence or stable housing for the millions of American women who suffer abuse. When we asked Francesca if she had ever gone to a battered women's shelter during the years that her ex-husband regularly beat her, she shrugged, "What was the point? They couldn't do anything." Battered women's shelters provide a temporary escape from a battering man, but are not positioned to solve the underlying problems of poverty and violence.[2] "How about reporting him to the police?" we asked. That was not even a possibility, Francesca explained, because Child Welfare Services could have used domestic violence as a reason to take her children away.

The dominant American paradigm according to which sexual violence is understood to be the aberrant actions of a single perpetrator against one or more specific victims cannot eliminate violence against women. Indeed, certain public policies, inadvertently or not, exacerbate the potential for violence. In response to police inaction regarding domestic violence, many states have passed mandatory arrest laws that require the police to arrest abusers when a domestic violence incident is reported. While this is a good idea in principle, women who report abuse risk further harm when violent men get a day or two in jail and come out even angrier and more likely to batter the women or their children (Davis, Weisburd, & Hamilton 2010; Iyengar 2007). Pouring salt on the wound, women who report abuse may find that they themselves are evicted from their homes. Vanessa, for instance, lost her government-subsidized housing because her violent and psychopathic former boyfriend stalked her. In the private housing sector, "nuisance" ordinances that sanction landlords for their tenants' behavior have been used to punish women for reaching out to the police for assistance. In Milwaukee, over a two-year period, nearly one-third of all nuisance citations were generated by domestic violence, and "most property owners 'abated' this nuisance by evicting battered women" (Desmond and Valdez 2012, p. 117). At least some, and possibly many, of these women end up homeless and thus even more vulnerable to violence and abuse.

———————

Although the United States has the highest incarceration rate in the world, the majority of those accused of rape are not arrested, and even when a rape charge is brought to court, the accused is often acquitted or pleads out for no jail time (Koss 2006). Of those accused, only an estimated 5 percent are convicted of rape, and only 3 percent spend any time in jail (cf. RAINN 2009). The National Violence against Women Survey (Tjaden & Thoennes 1998) analyzed 2,594 separate rape incidents among 8,000 female respondents. Of these 2,594 incidents, only 441 were reported to police, 33 were prosecuted, 13 resulted in convictions, and only 9 rapists were jailed. Data are scarce, but studies show that even in rape cases with biological evidence, such as matching semen or documentation of anogenital injury, less than a third of such cases made it to trial (Koss 2006).[3]

When women are frightened, bullied, or simply strung along into agreeing to lesser charges, and when the majority of rapists serve no jail time, there are spillover consequences for society. Every exonerated rapist (whether by the victim, her family, or the criminal justice system) fuels men and women's acceptance of the classic rape myths—that women often falsely accuse men of rape for revenge ("Hell hath no fury like a woman scorned") or to cover up their own promiscuous sexual activity. As a consequence of treating violence against women as individual acts of criminality, the character of the particular victim becomes relevant to the outcome of the case. Rape is one of the few crimes in which the victim is scrutinized for ulterior motives, false accusations, or signs of moral deviance. Victims least likely to see offenders convicted are older, are poorer, are deemed promiscuous or prostitutes, have a history of psychiatric diagnosis or drug abuse or a criminal record, did not overtly resist, were acquainted with the offender, or had a history of rape or abuse (Koss 2006).

Joy, a woman in her mid-thirties whom Francesca has tried to help, has bounced among the street, rehab facilities, and prison for more than a decade. Far less assertive and self-reliant than Francesca, Joy has not had a safe and stable place to live since she ran away from home as a teenager in the wake of sexual abuse. A few years after we met, she was brutally raped in her room in a "sober house" (housing for recovering addicts; we present more on Joy and on sober houses in chapter 6). When Joy went to court to testify against the rapist, the case against the perpetrator seemed ironclad. DNA evidence had led to his arrest originally—his DNA from a previous rape charge was found in the police computer system; police offers and crime scene officers testified; other witnesses from Joy's building testified; the emergency room nurse who examined her after the rape testified in court. However, the accused was found not guilty. Joy couldn't understand why. "The last three questions the defense attorney asked me are: Isn't it true that you were in prison? Isn't it true that you are an addict? Isn't it true that you used to work in prostitution?"[4]

While the notion that women who are victims of sexual or domestic violence bring their suffering on themselves is rarely declared aloud in twenty-first-century America, its currency is manifested through programs aimed at trying to reform or modify the victim's behaviors or attitudes. All of the Boston women, including Francesca, have been sent to therapeutic programs and spend many hours each week watching television shows that feature pop psychologists who explain the high rate of adult victimization of girls who grew up in abusive homes in terms of trauma that leads to poor self-esteem, emotional distress, and an unhealthy desire to harm oneself. Psychologically damaged by childhood sexual abuse, these poor, unhappy women are said to lack the sense of personal self-worth and autonomy believed necessary to avoid abusive relationships later in life (Van Bruggen, Runtz, & Kadlec 2006). This common wisdom, while kinder than older theories that saw abused women as liars, temptresses, or moral failures, still falls into the trap of stressing the character of the victim instead of the social forces that create situations of violence (cf. McKim 2008). In fact, *psychologists have come up with no consistent profile for women susceptible to domestic violence* (Herman 1997).

The messages conveyed by correctional, welfare, and therapeutic institutions link women's criminalization to their sexual victimhood; they are told that the same character flaws are the cause of both and that if they continue making bad choices they will continue being victims and they will continue being locked up. While victimhood may sometimes elicit sympathy, in much of mainstream American culture being a "victim" is denigrated as an indulgent choice, and "claims of victimization are scrutinized through a diagnostic lens as symptoms of impaired character rather than as matters of verifiable fact" (Cole 1999, p. 7). Victim blaming is made explicit when the victim is accused of having brought her suffering on herself by hanging out with the wrong crowd, wearing the wrong clothes, or going to the wrong places. Victim blaming takes a more subtle form when we publicly celebrate cancer survivors for battling against the disease, which may imply that those who do not survive—and who tend to be erased from public view—"gave up" or "fell victim to cancer." A corollary of victim blaming is the notion that one can refuse to be a victim, a claim suggesting that individuals have a choice in the matter. Indeed, blaming others for one's misfortunes is often seen as "an expression of weakness, moral or psychological, and a dangerous abdication of personal responsibility" (Cole 2007, p. 109).

The focus on the character flaws of individual perpetrators and victims obscures the structural inequalities that foster a great deal of the violence and suffering experienced by so many women and men. When hate-based violence is interpreted as idiosyncratic or aberrant rather than consistent with societal norms, resources are often poured into "correcting" victims through psychological treatment and into "correcting" perpetrators through penal treatment "rather than on dismantling the systemic forces that promote, condone, and facilitate . . . violence" (Mogul et al. 2011, p. 126).

———

Although only a small percentage of rapists and abusers serve substantial prison time, throughout the current age of mass incarceration millions of men have been thrown into jails and prisons in which the gender inequalities that underpin violence against women are intensified. In overcrowded jails, men and boys learn that in order to survive, they have to become "tough" and "numb to the pain of others" (Sabo, Kupers, & London 2001, p. 15; cf. Courtenay 2011, esp. p. 218). "Rape-based relationships between prisoners are often described as relationships between 'men' and 'girls' who are, in effect, thought of as 'master' and 'slave,' victor and vanquished" (Sabo 2001, p. 64). When men are released from prison, women easily become the targets of the rage, confusion, and exaggerated machismo that build up during incarceration. As Francesca told us one evening after Joey had spit on her, thrown the food she cooked out the window, and accused her of having sex with other men: "He has this man shit about him. Prison messed up his head. In jail people respected him—didn't mess with him. . . . He doesn't trust women."

FRANCESCA

After the surgery on her foot Francesca rested at her friend's apartment for a few weeks. But before her foot had fully healed, she decided she needed to start over with a clean slate: she would move to Florida to live with a man she had known years earlier. He sent her a bus ticket and picked her up at the station in Miami. Things were wonderful for a month or so while Francesca was passionately in love (according to posts she made several times each day on Facebook), but then "he told me he's not feeling it." Determined to stay off Percocet, she moved in with new friends she had made in the local Narcotics Anonymous community in Florida. These friends helped her find short-term jobs cleaning houses, painting, and waitressing. But after a few weeks her surgically treated foot began to throb. Not eligible for health insurance in Florida, she got on the bus and returned to Boston.

At the bus station we had trouble spotting her. No longer able to walk, she sat on top of her suitcase, hunched over in pain. By the time we arrived at the emergency room, her foot had swollen to twice its normal size and was bright red and oozing pus. Within ten minutes she was whisked back to surgery; the doctor later told us that she had come within hours of losing her foot. A week in the hospital provided Francesca rest, a respite from pain and homelessness, and a nice supply of her beloved Percocet. The day before she was to be released, she invited Joey to visit her. He seemed sullen, barely greeting us. But after we left, "I gave Joey a blow job," Francesca told us later. The next day she moved back in with him. A few days later her younger son joined them, and then a few months later her eldest son moved in as well. No longer in love with Joey but needing a place to stay, she sighed, "It is what it is. You do what you gotta do." A sentiment expressed by women around the world.

CHAPTER 2

"Nowhere to Go"

Poverty, Homelessness, and the Limits of Personal Responsibility

"I don't deserve to live like this. I'm not a bad person."

—Elizabeth

When one is looking for Elizabeth at any of the facilities and parks frequented by homeless Bostonians, the best bet is to ask for "the pretty blonde woman, about forty years old who is always crying." During the summer of 2008, Elizabeth spent most of her days in tears while wandering around the drop-in center carrying all of her belongings in an overflowing backpack. The first time we met her, we gave her five dollars so that she could rent a temporary locker at a homeless shelter. When we gave her the money, she wept even harder, choking out, "I have nowhere to go. My boyfriend just passed away. I was with him for six years. He passed away suddenly. He was healthy—he made me dinner the night before. We are waiting for the death certificate, the autopsy, to know why. I am heartbroken. I want to go to therapy but have to wait for an appointment. My support person is gone." Elizabeth sorrowfully speculated that she didn't know what to call herself now that her boyfriend was dead. She asked us if she was a widow. We told her yes. She seemed happy with that label as it validated her sense of loss. She never found out the official cause of death; his family refused to communicate with her.

During the next five years she would weep during almost every encounter or conversation, except when she was very drunk, during which times she could be quite jolly.

"My father was an alcoholic—although a beautiful man inside," Elizabeth mused. A police officer, he was accustomed to showing the world a domineering persona. Elizabeth's mother worked at a chemical company. "My mother wasn't able to show love. Maybe the chemicals are what caused her problems, her mental problems, and fibromyalgia." Elizabeth's father left when she was eleven. Several years later her mother married an emotionally abusive man. Following the family blueprint, Elizabeth's first boyfriend bossed her around. "He was my first love. I am always in abusive relationships—verbally or physically." Describing herself as a "whack job," Elizabeth explained that "both sides of my family have alcohol problems. It's genetic. Plus PTSD. My body doesn't produce serotonin and Neo-Synephrine."[1]

As a young woman Elizabeth was self-sufficient. She earned an associate's degree from a local college, always had her own apartment, and worked steadily in restaurant jobs. In some ways she was quite successful by mainstream American standards: she was self-supporting and even won a beauty pageant held for restaurant employees. And then, rather suddenly, when she was in her late twenties, Elizabeth was overwhelmed by a cascade of disasters beginning with the death of her older sister. "I held it in [the sadness], and it all came out when my sister died [of cancer]. She was a beautiful person; she never got mad at me if I did something wrong." "Like what?" we asked. Drawing on childhood memories, she replied, "Going into her room, touching her toys— kid things." Shortly after her sister died, Elizabeth's boss fired her for being "too depressed." Then, her apartment building was condemned for building code violations, and she had to move out. For the first time in her life Elizabeth became homeless. Reasonably resourceful at that point, she called her town hall for help and was told about the local homeless shelter. The rule at that shelter, as at many others, is that residents can stay for up to three months. At the end of her allotted time, feeling unable to manage on her own, Elizabeth moved in with a man she had met at the shelter. "He was an alcoholic and abusive," and it was this relationship, she believes, that thrust her into the world of homeless and alcoholic street people.

FROM THE WAR ON POVERTY TO THE WAR ON THE POOR

Poverty is not a fact of nature. In a country as blessed with natural resources as the United States, poverty is a consequence of choices we make as a society about how to distribute those resources. We all know about America's love affair with the self-sufficient hero who single-handedly overcomes all obstacles in *his* (sic) path. Certainly by long-held tradition, Americans have put their faith in the free market and in the notion that hard work is both morally laudable and a sure-fire path to personal success (Morone 2009). The forms in which these values are operationalized, however, and the fervor with which they are embraced change over time. In recent years income inequality has widened significantly (Jacobson & Occhino 2012); increasing numbers of Americans who want stable, full-time employment are stuck in low-wage, part-time, "revolving door" jobs (Cauthen 2011).

Most of the Boston women grew up in working-class households. Their parents came of age during the 1960s War on Poverty—named to denote a structural condition (poverty) and to call for structural solutions such as laws prohibiting racial bias in housing and employment. These parents worked throughout their adult lives at blue-collar jobs with decent wages, union contracts, health insurance, other benefits such as retirement pensions, and for bosses with some sense of loyalty toward their employees. Francesca and Elizabeth, on the other hand, came of age during a period of what has been called the War on the Poor. No longer working class, they are what is known as the working poor; that is, increasingly marginalized Americans who work at jobs without benefits, security, or adequate work safety provisions; jobs that do not pay sufficiently to allow one to rise out of poverty; jobs without the kind of informal social contract that would induce an employer to carry a worker like Elizabeth for a few weeks while she could recover from a family tragedy.

The policies that created this state of affairs are known collectively as Reaganomics or neoliberalism: a set of principles the include minimal government involvement in the economy; the notion of "trickle down" wealth distribution (the idea that when the rich thrive, prosperity trickles down to middle- and low-income people); tax laws that favor the wealthy through loopholes and other exemptions of various kinds; de-unionizing of labor forces; privatization in areas such as health care, energy distribution, and prisons; and deregulation of industry and trade. Free-trade agreements that encourage outsourcing of jobs to states and countries where wages are low and where the manufacturing costs are lower because of, among other factors, weaker worker safety provisions have hit families like Elizabeth's particularly hard.

Although the roots of neoliberalism go back at least two hundred years, it was during the Reagan era of the 1980s that the United States adopted many of the specific policies that have created our current, radically unequal society. Quite simply, more and more people are becoming poor, remaining poor, and raising children in poverty. Women in particular bear the burdens of neoliberal economic policies. According to the Bureau of Labor Statistics (2013), women who usually worked full-time in 2012 had median weekly earnings of $692, or 79.1 percent of the $875 weekly median for men. Nearly half of the difference between female and male poverty rates is explained by the preponderance of women in the three lowest-wage occupations—food preparation and serving, cleaning and maintenance, and personal care and service— occupational sectors with particularly low rates of unionization (Lichtenwalter 2005).

When Elizabeth first became unemployed, she did what many Americans would think to do: she applied for welfare. Almost immediately, an employee at the Department of Transitional Assistance (the welfare office) told her that since she was a single woman with no children, her application for welfare would not be accepted. Although Elizabeth did not know this at the time, Congress in 1996 had passed the Personal Responsibility and Work Opportunity Act (PRWORA, commonly called "welfare reform"), which, as President Bill Clinton proudly proclaimed at the time, "end[ed] welfare as we know it." PRWORA eliminated the safety net that had been provided for chronically poor families by Aid to Families with Dependent Children, and replaced it with Temporary Assistance to Needy Families (TANF), a program that sets strict limits on the lifetime number of years (five) an individual can receive assistance. The name *Temporary* Assistance to Needy *Families* (TANF) underscores both the provisional, short-term nature of our nation's primary program for providing cash benefits to the poor, and which poor people (families only) are considered worthy of receiving those benefits. As a society we may be willing to support innocent children who are poor "through no fault of their own," but we are not willing to provide financial assistance to adults (who, it is often assumed, are at fault for being poor).

The very title of the act enunciated the ideology of welfare reform: rather than making welfare the responsibility of society to care for vulnerable members, PRWORA cast poverty as a personal matter. The moralistic rhetoric surrounding the passage of PRWORA emphasized the character traits of poor people: bad attitudes, an inadequate sense of personal responsibility, and a deficient work ethic. The policies that govern and manage the poor have less to do with transforming the conditions that lead to poverty and more to do with efforts to "transform the poor themselves—to make them into the kinds of subjects who voluntarily embrace particular kinds of choices and behaviors" (Soss, Fording, & Schram 2012, p. 9). With no more than a gentle kick in the behind, the argument went, welfare mothers would find that they actually can support themselves—and would develop self-esteem and a stronger backbone by doing so. Welfare, it was said, is a disincentive to work, and welfare dependency leads to crime and out-of-wedlock births (Weaver & Duongtran 2009). Over the past few decades welfare dependency has been medicalized by identifying it as a pathology similar to a chemical addiction. "Welfare programs, in this frame, follow a 'recovery model' that is closely aligned with the twelve-step programs. . . . Through the lens of the recovery model, welfare recipients are cast as disordered subjects who require a transformative program to cure their pathologies and help them gain control over their lives" (Soss, Fording, & Schram 2012, pp. 241–242).

In line with the personal responsibility mantra, job-training programs are the centerpiece of PRWORA. These programs typically emphasize individual flaws (e.g., that women need to adopt a proper work ethic and to learn "how to be an employee," how to wake up to go to a job), rather than the economic reality of high rates of unemployment and the harsh conditions and instability of low-wage work. While most of the Boston women have participated in multiple job-training programs, only one actually landed a steady job at the end. More typical was the job-training program Tonya went through: she was given a mop and broom and assigned to clean the building in which the program's offices are located. She was paid $8 an hour and worked three hours a day. The program lasted for one month, during which time her caseworker was supposed to try to find her a real job. At the end of the "training" she was not placed into a job, an outcome for which Tonya blames the caseworker and the caseworker attributes to the poor economy and Tonya's "attitude." This is a routine that Tonya knows well. Over the years we have known her she has been sent to several rounds of training in food service. Typically the "training" consisted of being sent to do low-level kitchen work in a hotel or a government cafeteria. Alongside job-training programs Tonya has participated in numerous anger management classes and parenting classes. "I feel like I'm in a loop of doing program after program but not getting anywhere."

Despite rhetoric regarding the family as the cornerstone of American society (and the word *family* in the very title of TANF), institutional policies often pit women and men against each other. Women may risk losing their public housing, welfare, and food stamps when a man—even her children's father—is caught living in her apartment. Exacerbating matters for poor women, PRWORA allows states to impose family caps on the receipt of additional cash benefits when the birth of a child increases the size of a family. The family cap rule is particularly harmful in regions of the country where low-income women cannot access birth control and where there are few or no abortion providers. The rule also disadvantages women who do not believe that abortion is ethical and women whose sexual partners prevent them from seeking abortions. Since more than half of women receiving welfare benefits have been victims of male violence, the family cap seems unnecessarily punitive (Richie 2012, p. 115).

———

The United States spends around $75 billion dollars annually on imprisonment (Schmitt, Warner, & Gupta, 2010), a figure far higher than the $32 billion spent annually on TANF (Urban Institute 2012). The average monthly remittance for a welfare recipient family was $392 in fiscal year 2010 (Office of Family Assistance 2012). However, according to the Massachusetts Economic Independence Index, the monthly income necessary for one adult to afford basic necessities, including housing, utilities, food, basic transportation, health care, basic clothing, essential personal and household items, and taxes, in the Boston area is $2,375 (Ames et al. 2013). Because welfare payments are not sufficient for rent, utilities, transportation, and items not covered by food stamps (such as toilet paper, toothpaste, and soap), TANF recipients may rely on homeless shelters or supplement their allowance through shoplifting or other nonlegal behavior that may lead to involvement with the correctional system (Butcher & LaLonde 2006; Hays 2003). As one might expect, women's incarceration rates go down when welfare payments go up (Heimer et al. 2012).

The stinginess of welfare payments is intended to make being on welfare uncomfortable. Welfare recipients are required to certify and recertify their eligibility and prove that there is no man living with them (a co-resident man is assumed to be bringing in money). Being on welfare exposes women to institutional surveillance to ensure that they actively seek employment but do not earn "too much" money, and that they do not receive financial support from a family member or male partner. Our national obsession with so-called welfare fraud has engendered an institutionalized hypervigilance and suspicion that seem completely unrelated to the miserable reality of the day-to-day lives of poor Americans. We Americans seem terrified, or enraged, at the possibility that someone will cheat or "pull one over" on us. Thus, women like Elizabeth need to put in a great deal of work to prove to the appropriate gate-keepers and policy makers that they are truly "needy," that they are not trying to trick the government into giving them something that they do not deserve. But given the undesirable traits associated with "neediness" in American culture, need-based responses to suffering slide into punitive and carceral responses—what we have called the dual-sided coin of medicalization and criminalization.

THE POLITICS OF DISABILITY

Ineligible for welfare, Elizabeth began the process of applying for Social Security Disability Insurance (SSDI), the federal insurance program for workers who have become disabled. At the Social Security office she was told that to apply for SSDI she would need a doctor's report documenting that she is too mentally ill to work. With a sleight of the bureaucratic hand, Elizabeth's suffering, which had resulted from economic policies, was recast as personal pathology. With a doctor's letter attesting to her bipolar disorder and PTSD (caused, as she explained to us, by the assaults experienced while homeless), she submitted her application. It was denied, as was her appeal. Although nothing changed in the interim, on her third appeal she was granted SSDI benefits of approximately $850 per month. Her experiences were typical. Throughout the country approximately two-thirds of disability cases are not accepted when first filed, though the majority of rejections are eventually overturned when taken to court; two-thirds of those who appeal an initial rejection eventually win their cases (Eckholm 2007). Although Elizabeth had worked and paid into Social Security throughout the first decades of her adult life, the application and appeal process made it clear to her that basic financial resources are not a *right* to which she is entitled by virtue of being a human being. Rather, to receive even minimal help, she had to demonstrate to the satisfaction of doctors and bureaucrats that she is truly *needy*.

Elizabeth is lucky: she is the only one of the Boston woman who qualifies for SSDI. More than half of the women receive Supplemental Security Income (SSI), the American safety net for disabled adults and children who have limited income and resources but do not qualify for SSDI because they have not worked a sufficient number of years for employers who paid into Social Security. (For a forty-year-old this would be approximately ten years). As of December 2012, the number of SSI recipients was about 8.3 million. The average monthly SSI payment was $519, and most recipients had no income other than their monthly SSI remittance. Six out of ten SSI recipients under age sixty-five have been diagnosed with a mental disorder, and the majority (about 54 percent) of recipients are women (U.S. Social Security Administration 2013). While we recognize that SSI and SSDI payments constitute the difference between scraping by and utter destitution for millions of Americans, we find it disturbing that such large numbers of people (especially women) are certified as too mentally ill to work. These numbers suggest either that American culture is literally making people sick or that millions of Americans submit to being labeled mentally ill in order to receive the $519 per month that barely allows them to afford minimal food and housing. In Elizabeth's case both were true. The ongoing stresses and stigmas of poverty and sexual assault caused her health to deteriorate. At the same time, she had few choices other than to adopt the status "disabled" in order to obtain financial assistance.

In that regard, Elizabeth resembles many other Americans. Following PROWRA's enactment the number of Americans on welfare declined at approximately the same rate at which the number of Americans on SSI and SSDI increased. One would expect medical advances to have reduced the numbers of disabled children and adults; but in fact, every month 14 million people now get a disability check from the government. As Chana Joffe-Walt argued in a report for National Public Radio (2013), SSI and SSDI have turned into the de facto safety net for Americans unable to find steady employment that pays a living wage:

> People who leave the workforce and go on disability qualify for Medicare, the government health care program that also covers the elderly. They also get disability payments from the government of about $13,000 a year. This isn't great. But if your alternative is a minimum wage job that will pay you at most $15,000 a year, and probably does not include health insurance, disability may be a better option. But, in most cases, going on disability means you will not work, you will not get a raise, you will not get whatever meaning people get from work. Going on disability means, assuming you rely only on those disability payments, you will be poor for the rest of your life. That's the deal. And it's a deal 14 million Americans have signed up for." (Joffe-Walt 2013)

By labeling certain people or groups as needy or disabled, we define them as weak, as victims, as lacking in the attributes that our society admires, and as having physical or emotional flaws that, with the right balance of education and punishment, will be rectified (cf. Blackwell 1999). Sentiments of this sort were infamously articulated in 2012 when presidential candidate Mitt Romney chastised the "47 percent of Americans who will automatically vote for Obama. . . . [These are people] who are dependent upon government, who believe that they are victims, who believe the government has a responsibility to care for them, who believe that they are entitled to health care, to food, to housing, to you-name-it . . . that that's an entitlement and the government should give it to them. . . . These are people who pay no income tax." Romney condemned victims on two counts: they do not contribute to the greater good of society ("pay no income tax"), and they may well be making false claims ("believe that they are victims").

ELIZABETH

In the winter of 2009 rumors floated around the women's center that Elizabeth was in the hospital. When we stopped by to visit with flowers and chocolate, she was a bit doped up on Percocet, but still lucid enough to tell us that she had fallen while trying to climb over a wall with her heavy pack on her back. She mostly wanted to talk about her anxiety regarding where she would go "when they make me leave the hospital." Unable to bear any weight on her ankle, which would be in a cast for the next six weeks, she could not go back to the streets or the shelters. She also didn't want to go to a nursing home with "people who are old and dying and incontinent."

At the last minute, hospital employees found a bed for her at a respite facility for the homeless. It was a clean and well-run facility in terms of medical treatment, but the downside for Elizabeth was that "they don't allow residents to leave at all. It felt like jail," she told us. Chafing at being treated like a prisoner for the crime of being homeless and injured, Elizabeth stayed for only one month. Back on the shelter circuit, Elizabeth now had to deal with a new set of problems. Because of her ankle surgery she needed a bottom bunk bed but could not request one without a doctor's note. However, if she were to get the necessary doctor's note, she could be turned away from the shelter completely if there was no bottom bunk available. Taking whatever she could get, most nights she struggled into a top bunk. Making matters worse, her SSDI checks had stopped coming. It turned out that in the chaos of the surgery and the moves, she had neglected to return the "twenty-page form" needed to recertify her SSDI eligibility. Although Elizabeth blamed her own "procrastination," the recertification process actually involves actions by a number of people, including her psychiatrist, who needed to fax various documents to the Social Security office but apparently neglected to do so. In the meantime she resorted to panhandling (she called it "stemming") for change. Eventually Elizabeth found a shelter caseworker to help her complete the recertification process. By the time her ankle healed, however, Elizabeth was barred from the shelter for two weeks for having taken a shower after lights-out. (Elizabeth often has trouble being assertive enough to get time in the showers during the hours allotted.) She decided not to go to the other large women's shelter in Boston. "The staff and the women there are mean. There is no respect, the way they treat me. I'm afraid that I'll blow up and end up in even more trouble." Elizabeth's concerns were justified. A few months later we met her at the emergency room, where she was told she needed surgery for a deviated septum. It turned out that a woman at a shelter had punched Elizabeth in the nose because she had talked to the woman's boyfriend.

Shortly after that emergency room visit Elizabeth was lucky enough to win the lottery for a two-month reserved bed at a shelter that allows women to stay inside during the day. "I am blessed to have this bed," Elizabeth told us. "I can do what I like, read, rest, and they have activities. I made Christmas ornaments." This shelter, however, is especially strict, enforcing numerous rules concerning the daily schedule, resident behavior, and guest interactions that are easily violated. Of the approximately twenty women who had started with Elizabeth, only six remained after a month. Some left voluntarily; others were asked to leave because of infractions that included using "bad" language (swear words), arguing with other guests or with staff members, and forgetting to put on plastic gloves before taking a snack from the refrigerator. Elizabeth lasted about six weeks.

THE INSTITUTIONAL CIRCUIT

In looking back through our notes, we were surprised to see how much public assistance Elizabeth received over the years of the project. Despite that assistance—and despite the genuine goodwill of nearly all of the caseworkers and other helpers we have met—the agencies and programs on the institutional circuit far too rarely attained the professed goals of keeping people healthy, helping those with financial troubles get back on their feet, rehabilitating "offenders," or deterring crime (cf. Mulia 2002).

The institutional circuit, while quite cohesive in ideological matters, is mind-bogglingly fragmented in terms of day-to-day functioning (cf. Sered & Norton-Hawk 2013). Emergency assistance programs make frequent changes in eligibility criteria for those seeking services. Homeless shelters have rules that make no sense for the population that utilizes shelters. Programs start with good intentions and then close because funding is withdrawn or priorities change. Facilities and caseworkers do not communicate with one another, clients need to fill out multiple forms and chase down numerous documents from various providers, and the duration of service provision often seems unrelated to the need the service is supposed to fill. (Time limits on stays at homeless shelters are an obvious example; one-week drug treatment programs another.) Within facilities caseworkers and providers come and go, burned out by the challenges of the population with which they are charged to work, underpaid, and frequently laid off when funding is cut. While criminalized women in Massachusetts rarely have to forgo medical treatment because of an inability to pay (Massachusetts has near-universal health care coverage), the services available to them tend to be disjointed, partial, and short-term. Each woman circulates among dozens of providers at multiple facilities; tests are done, but treatment plans are not executed; and short-term psychotherapy opens wounds but rarely brings about any feeling of closure. Like Elizabeth, the women we have come to know find that they need to put in a lot of work in order to receive the support and the services that, in most other industrialized countries, are considered a basic human right.

The inadequacy of safety net services seems designed to operate as a kick in the pants that will push the needy person into becoming a "productive citizen." However, policies and practices often keep women like Elizabeth captive on the institutional circuit. Because SSI and TANF remittances are not sufficient to live on, recipients turn to homeless shelters or other housing programs, the correctional system, or dependence on men that may well lead to dependence on battered women's and victims' assistance programs. For a mother, residence in a homeless shelter is a surefire way to involve Child Welfare Services. CWS is more likely than not to send women to various therapeutic programs as well as drug-testing programs, which in turn readily lock women into the correctional system. Children drawn into Child Welfare Services are more likely than other children to end up in juvenile detention facilities, jails, and prisons. And the best predictor for incarceration is having been incarcerated in the past (Nieto 2002).

The humiliations, hassles, and suspicion directed at those seeking public services speak clearly to the lower status of "the needy" in a society that valorizes strength and autonomy. We have come to understand that while the failures of the institutional circuit to effectively address suffering often look as if they are merely bureaucratic, the medium is in fact the message that the real problem lies with the individual, not the collective, and public agencies are not the answer to human affliction in this era of neoliberal governance. We make this point in order to defuse the idea that, even with the best intentions, doctors, police, therapy, day programs, soup kitchens, anger management classes, and rehabilitation centers cannot eliminate the suffering caused by structural violence and by economic, gender, and racial inequalities.

"IN THE HOMELESS LIFE"

Elizabeth told us that she feels she can deal with being poor, but what "does me in" is homelessness. When she first became homeless, Elizabeth did not know that she should get on the waiting list for public housing and for Section VIII government housing subsidies (a voucher program that helps low-income Americans pay rent). By the time she learned about those programs, she was no longer eligible because of her record of incarceration for offenses including public intoxication, an offense that in and of itself was a function of being homeless. (If she had still had her apartment, she would likely not have been drinking in the Boston Common.)

Elizabeth is also adamant that she is not a "homeless person" but rather "in the homeless life." This distinction clarifies that homelessness is not a character trait but rather a product of economic systems in which certain people own property and others do not. According to the Homelessness Research Institute (2012), the average real income of working-poor Americans in 2010 was $9,400. "There was not a single county in the nation," the study found, "where a family with an average annual income of $9,400 could afford fair market rent for a one-bedroom unit" (p. 4). "Over the course of a year," the HRI report continues, "the estimated odds of experiencing homelessness are approximately 1 in 194 for the general population, though the odds vary by circumstance. The odds of experiencing homelessness for people with incomes at or below the federal poverty line have increased to an estimated 1 in 29" (p. 38). Boston is among the top seven most expensive rental areas in the country, with a median gross monthly rent of $1,162 (U.S. Census Bureau

2012). There are federal, state, and municipal housing programs aimed at moving homeless Americans into housing, but funding for these programs is chronically insufficient. In place of policies that address structural issues related to the cost of housing, most U.S. cities use temporary shelters as the primary means for getting the homeless off the streets. And even the best and largest local homeless programs are neither mandated nor funded to address the economic conditions that push people into homelessness.

Staying at shelters has been difficult for Elizabeth on many levels. Her misery in the shelters stems from several sources, including the numerous rules regarding such things as bathroom use; her weepy affect, which, unfortunately, makes her vulnerable to stronger and more assertive shelter residents; and tough requirements regarding shelter entry. Other residents often bully her, and when she fights back, she ends up being barred by shelters for getting into arguments. She indignantly explains that "there is . . . no respect. I have constant panic attacks and anxiety." At most shelters anyone wanting a bed has to arrive by 2:30 in the afternoon, a requirement that makes it difficult for Americans dependent upon shelters to go to doctors' appointments, job interviews, or even other government agencies. Arriving on time at a shelter does not guarantee a bed. "My heart is in my mouth every day because they have a lottery." Each woman requesting a bed for the night is given a number. A staff member puts the numbers into a bowl and picks about seventy women out of the ninety who come on an average day. "It's like playing bingo," she says. When we asked, "What do you do when you aren't lucky?" she replied, "I just sit there and say I have no place to go. About 9:30 at night they bring out a cot for me, but then they wake me up at 4:30 in the morning." Guests in regular beds are woken at 6:00.

Shelter guests typically cannot leave their belongings at the shelter during the day when the facility is closed. The obligation to carry her possessions with her when she leaves early each morning makes Elizabeth vulnerable to theft. Elizabeth has had all of her belongings, including her medication, stolen several times. Many of the better shelters in the Boston area (i.e., those that have beds and blankets rather than simply floor space for sleeping) prohibit entry to people who are visibly drunk or high (a policy that makes little sense given the number of homeless people who use drugs or alcohol) and limit stays to five days, two weeks, or one month. Instead of settling down in one place and getting organized, Elizabeth starts over with a new caseworker each time she moves to another shelter—a process that is both emotionally painful when old wounds are reopened in the retelling, and logistically wasteful when caseworkers duplicate applications and services.

Rules requiring shelter residents to leave early each morning are intended to encourage homeless people to go out and look for work.[2] While shelter employees generally understand that most residents are unemployable, the strict timetables are maintained as part of the larger regimen of shaping the homeless into normative—that is, self-sufficient—American citizens. "I don't deserve all the bad things that happen to me," Elizabeth told us. "I'm confused. I'm trying to go down the right path, but the tide is going against me. . . . I just make stupid mistakes. I miss appointments. I'm a procrastinator, an idiot. I get off the bus at the wrong place. I don't have any structure. Especially being homeless, I don't even have a place to write things down." Shuffling through a pile of paper scraps with phone numbers for therapeutic programs, addresses of places to get lunch, and dates and times of appointments with caseworkers, Elizabeth—in a rare moment of good humor—joked, "Homelessness is a full time job."

————

Mental illness—or, more specifically, the greater number of mentally ill thought to be on the streets because of the deinstitutionalization of state mental hospitals in the 1960s—is often blamed for the "epidemic" of homelessness. In fact, however, rates of homelessness in U.S. cities skyrocketed during the 1980s when conservative economic and social welfare policies led more and more Americans into poverty while the cost of housing rose and the availability of rental housing declined. Although it certainly is the case that many mentally ill people become homeless, deinstitutionalized former patients actually constitute a small percentage of homeless Americans (Mathieu 1993). For many homeless people, it is living on the street that causes psychological and physical distress (National Coalition for the Homeless 2009).

Without housing it is difficult for one to maintain the kind of outward appearance that makes one employable. Homeless shelters, while better than the street in most cases, are epidemiological pumps. With beds crammed together, viruses, infections, anxiety, and exhaustion lead residents into clinics and hospitals. Researchers in Boston found that 119 persons who experienced chronic homelessness for five years running (1999–2003) made more than 18,000 emergency room visits (Mangano 2007).[3] Crowded shelters with bunk beds clustered close together and shared bathroom facilities provide fertile breeding grounds for colds, flu, and MRSA (multidrug-resistant *Staphylococcus aureus*, which has become the bane of hospitals, barracks, and homeless shelters). The free meals at shelters and soup kitchens tend to be served in crowded halls, rushed, and heavy on processed meats. On numerous occasions we lined up with Elizabeth or Francesca an hour or more before lunch in order to be served a plate of hot dogs and canned corn. Like many other Americans, homeless people soothe hunger pangs with cigarettes, soda pop, and whatever snack food in an extra-large package is on sale at the local convenience store.

When insecurely housed, women in particular are at heightened risk of assault. In a Florida study, Jasinski and colleagues (2010) found that one in four homeless women is homeless mainly because of her experiences with violence and that, in a vicious cycle, leaving a violent partner put women at risk for violence on the streets. Filling out the cycle, homeless people are more likely to be stopped and arrested, which then—as happened to Elizabeth— results in losing one's eligibility for public housing and government housing subsidies (chapter 8 discusses barriers to housing and government services faced by former inmates). To get a clearer sense of what life is like in the home-less shelters at night, we sat down with several of the caseworkers at one of the larger shelters for women in the Boston area. "Ambulances come here almost every night, most often for people who are having seizures," one case-worker told us. The seizures are caused by complications stemming from psychiatric medication, drug overdoses, diabetes, and head trauma. The case-workers told us that for women more than men, living on the streets causes mental illness. "The women here age quickly—many of them are walking with canes even at an early age." In any given year, homeless Americans are three to four times more likely to die than those with housing; the mortality rates of homeless women ages eighteen to thirty-five is as high as thirty-one times that of housed women in the same age cohort (O'Connell 2005).

ELIZABETH

When spring returned to Boston, Elizabeth went back to sleeping in the Boston Common. One night a man she had been acquainted with ("a drinking buddy") kicked her in the face and sexually assaulted her. The police came, caught him red-handed with her pocketbook, and took her to the emergency room. Terrified, in pain, with her face covered with blood, she was asked if she wanted a rape kit done. Since there was no penetration (he pulled down her pants and rubbed himself on her), Elizabeth mistakenly assumed that that the rape kit would be of no use. In any case, she was more concerned at that moment about the blood dripping down her face and could not even think about a rape kit.

Elizabeth hoped the police would lock up her attacker and "throw away the key." But when we ran into her a few weeks later, she told us that the court-appointed victim's advocate had informed her that because the court calendar was full, her attacker was going to be tried in a lower court where the maximum sentence is two and a half years. Elizabeth was also told that she would have to testify and that the defense attorney would most likely tear her apart on the stand because of her prison record. Over the next few months she went to court at least three times, spending entire days sitting and waiting for the case to be heard. When she complained, the judge yelled at her and threatened to put an arrest warrant out on *her* if she did not come back for the next court date. In the end her attacker served a short sentence for assault and battery.

A few months later, on a night when she couldn't get a bed at one of the larger shelters, Elizabeth went to sleep on a bench at a train station. She had come to feel that it was too dangerous to sleep in more open places like parks where, she explained, "people are murdered all the time." She was arrested for trespassing on the station grounds by a police officer who "doesn't like homeless people." In court for the trespassing charges, she was ordered to pay a $300 fine. She did not have the money. Exasperated, she noted, "This is a waste of the court's time . . . they should be going after real criminals."

Like many homeless men and women, Elizabeth likes to spring for a couple of nights in a motel when she receives her Social Security check. This is her only opportunity to sleep in a room not shared with dozens of other women, to read in bed as late as she likes, to sleep late in the morning, and to stay inside during the day. So, about six months after the rape, Elizabeth sought a night's refuge in a motel. In the morning when she went to check out, the motel clerk would not return her $50 room deposit; he said he would mail it to her later in the week. "It was my money. He was supposed to give it to me. I can't wait for the money, I have nothing. I think he was trying to cheat me, so I called the police." When the police came they looked at her ID, saw that she owed the $300 fine, and arrested and handcuffed her. "I spent three days in jail waiting for a judge because it was a three-day weekend."

Not long afterward Elizabeth was shoved to the floor by a man she was staying with. Both intoxicated and reeling from her head having hit the floor, she grabbed a knife in self-defense. However, the man got hold of it and gashed her finger open. When Elizabeth arrived at the emergency room inebriated and disgruntled, the staff notified the police. When the officers arrived, they looked her up and saw that she was out on bail for a previous charge. Panicked and still inebriated, she was deemed to be engaged in disorderly conduct, which constituted noncompliance with the conditions of her bail. She was sent to the Massachusetts Correctional Institution for sixty days. "I was stabbed and almost lost my finger. They stitched it up and then sent me to prison."

Elizabeth's run of bad luck convinced her to go back to the shelters. She reluctantly began shuttling between a shelter she liked that has a policy of six days residence followed by four days out, and another shelter she does not like because residents have to be upstairs in the sleeping area by 6:00 p.m., showered and in pajamas by 8:00, under lights-out by 10:00, up at 6:00 a.m., and downstairs dressed and ready for breakfast by 6:30. After a few months of shelter shuffle Elizabeth thought she had finally hit the jackpot. A bed was found for her in a small, two-year residential program for homeless women living with mental health challenges. Although this facility provided a guaranteed bed and an alcohol/drug counselor, it closed its doors during the day, leaving the women to fend for themselves. One morning while Elizabeth was napping in a secluded corner of a local train station, a man who had followed her beat her about the head, choked her, ripped off her pants, underwear and shoes, and tried to rape her. Wearing only her shirt, she managed to get away and flagged down a passing bus. When we visited her at the same respite facility where she had gone to recover after her ankle surgery, she was in tears. "Only by the grace of God I got away," she repeated to us as well as to every person who came into her room.

In 2011, with the help of a caseworker, Elizabeth successfully appealed her disqualification for public housing and Section VIII vouchers. But when the caseworker signed her up for the lottery for an apartment in Boston Public Housing, she was told it could take as long as ten years for her name to be drawn. Section VIII eligibility proved equally useless; on her Social Security Disability check of approximately $845 per month Elizabeth could not find an apartment that she could afford in the Boston area in a building willing to rent to a Section VIII tenant. The caseworker explained to us that many landlords assume that Section VIII tenants will cause problems. While the caseworker could move mountains of paperwork, she could not manipulate the housing market or a cultural ethos that blames the poor for being poor.

A year or so later Elizabeth disappeared for a while from the shelter circuit, the women's center, and the Boston Common. And then, out of the blue, four months before this writing, she stopped by our office to apologize for not having been in touch. Sobbing when we gave her the mass-transit pass that all of the project participants are entitled to receive monthly, she told us, "You are so nice to me and I don't deserve it. I'm a whack job."

CHAPTER 3

"The Little Rock of the North"

Race, Gender, Class, and the Consequences of Mass Incarceration

[Black] women actually experience various forms of violence as layers of degradation that have a cumulative negative effect on their lives, resulting in systematic subordination.

—Beth E. Richie, *Arrested Justice* (2012)

Despite differences created by historical era, age, social class, sexual orientation, skin color, or ethnicity, the legacy of struggle against the violence that permeates U.S. social structures is a common thread binding African-American women.

—Patricia Hill Collins, *Black Feminist Thought* (2000)

When Anasia walks into the drop-in center, a few of the more timid women show a sudden need to leave for a cigarette, a bathroom run, or a vague appointment. Younger women may jump up to steer her to the most comfortable chair in the room, where she plops down with a thump and a groan. A heavy-set black woman in her late thirties, Anasia walks with a limp, listing to one side like a boat missing a rudder. Known for her street smarts and her quick temper, she is proud to have done whatever she needed to do to survive, and is not reticent when talking about shoplifting, selling drugs, or using other people to get what she needs. Many of the project participants prefer to shield us from direct knowledge of their illegal activities. In contrast, shortly after we first met Anasia, she stopped by our office asking if we had a plastic bag we could give her. "I picked up a couple of things and they are making my pockets looked stuffed," she explained in a nonchalant tone of voice as she pulled out four bottles of men's shampoo that she had just stolen from a store across the street.

————

Chaos is Anasia's word of choice for describing her family, her neighborhood, and her life. As a child, she and her siblings bounced between the house of their functioning but alcoholic mother and their father, an "abuser and serial cheater." Outside the house, things were no better. "I was moving from school to school, from place to place—it was crazy. When we first moved [to the Boston housing projects]," Anasia recalls, "it was more white people than black people; there were only like five black people, so they used to stone our house and write 'Get out nigger' on the doors and windows and stuff. And stuff like that, take our bikes, and stuff like that . . . I mean, we weathered the storm and we got through that, and then it got mixed."

During the 1970s when Anasia was growing up, Boston earned the nickname the "Little Rock of the North." In 1974, federal district court judge Arthur Garrity, Jr. found the Boston School Committee (the city's board of education) guilty of enforcing segregation in its schools. As a result, a mandated program of busing white students to predominantly black schools and black students to predominantly white schools was instituted. In retrospect this attempt at desegregation was modest in size. At the time, however, fights and riots broke out at South Boston High, Hyde Park High, and Charlestown High in opposition to busing. Within the first twenty-six days of the school year, there were over 140 arrests and reports of sixty-nine treatable injuries (Formisano 1991, p. 80). The tenacity of black parents determined to send their children to better schools reflects both personal courage and the abominable state of the segregated black schools of the time. Jonathan Kozol (1985), who taught in a school in Boston's primarily black Roxbury neighborhood in 1964, documented peeling paint, lack of textbooks, underqualified teachers, and overcrowded classrooms. Even more damning, he wrote, "the slave-master and black child feeling was prevalent" (p. 41).

Anasia recalls that school was a struggle for her. "It wasn't going real well. I mean every time I'd make friends, we was up and moving, leaving, going somewhere else, and then I had to make friends all over again and it was like chaos. Constant chaos. . . . One of my friends was smoking weed at that age [twelve], so [I started smoking] in order to fit in." Kicked out of the regular public school, she "started going to whatever they call the school for bad people." She dropped out when she was sixteen, "and I didn't have to go no more." No one seemed to make an effort to bring her back in to school.

Anasia's first boyfriend was a drug dealer, "so I no longer had to pay for [crack cocaine]. I always had it, right there." With her boyfriend she had two children. Reluctant to leave her crack supplier, Anasia frequently turned to her mother for support when her children's father hurt her or when he went to jail. "When I had my oldest son, immediately my mother took him because my mother said, 'I'd be damned if he beat my grandson.'" Her mother remained the primary caregiver of her elder son; her sister the primary caregiver of the younger. "I just went off . . . into the world. Doing what I wanted to do, constantly going to jail. I would only call my mother when I went to jail so she could send me some canteen money." Over the years Anasia has had other boyfriends, who "did the same things I did. Stole, went to jail. Bad boys, all of them."

INTERSECTIONS OF RACE AND GENDER, PART I

In chapter 1 we describe gender overdetermination as a social process in which femaleness is always made relevant, in which diverse social attributes are explained in terms of physical gender, in which gender trumps personhood. Parallel processes (though not parallel content) describe the persistent salience of race and racism in America (Bonilla-Silva 2013). For black women like Anasia, these potent social processes intersect: she is never "only" a woman or "only" African American. Both gender and race shape her engagements with family, community, employers, doctors, welfare institutions, and the correctional system.[1]

Like Francesca, nearly all of the white project participants narrated a path to pain, homelessness, and criminalization that revolved around childhood sexual abuse followed by PTSD and drug use. As their lives spiraled downward, many of the white women were cut off by their natal families for reasons ranging from well-intentioned "tough love," meant to bring the daughter to her senses, to exasperation, fear, and shame. In the words of one white parent we talked to, "She grew up with everything, but she acts like she comes from the ghetto."

Most of the black women in the Boston group grew up in "respectable" poor families; they may have lived in the housing projects, but their parents worked and managed to scrape by. While some of the black women were sexually abused as children, most recalled growing up in supportive house-holds and continued to maintain positive relationships with their families (see Richie 1996). Even Anasia, whose father molested her, felt that her mother had always been there for her. Though disappointed when Anasia, as she puts it, "messes up," her mother would never consider *not* helping her out. According to the family ethos, Anasia explained, you help and protect other family members when they are in trouble. Indeed, Anasia's family has remained mutually supportive—providing one another a place to stay, taking care of one another's children, making efforts to keep one another safe, and helping one another deal with government agencies. Her eldest son, now in his twenties, has become her protector. "He smokes weed. . . . That's one thing I never hid from my oldest son. Like when I was getting high and he was younger, he knew, you know what I'm saying? I would tell him. . . . And I think he respects me more because of that." Over the past few years her son has taken on the responsibility to come and get her when she runs into trouble in a crack house. "My son takes care of me. He will go to the crack house with me and make sure I get out of there. He doesn't use, but watches out for me. People are scared of him and they know they shouldn't mess with him."

For the black women we met, far more than for the white women, it was the outside world more than the domestic one that set them onto a path of suffering. Vanessa was raised by warm and loving parents in the 1960s in a segregated black neighborhood where much of the housing was contaminated with high levels of lead. As a result of childhood lead poisoning, she struggles with reading, memory, and an array of other cognitive challenges. Mary, a black woman in her early fifties, explains that she and some other black students would be passed to the next grade in school even if they couldn't read, because they were needed on the track team. Given no remedial help (though plenty of track team coaching), Mary finished high school unable to fill out job application forms.

While most of the white women eagerly share psychologically framed narratives tracing their drug use to trauma, Anasia expresses little interest in picking apart her intrapsychic motivations. "There is no particular reason—I just do it. I seem to be doing good [not using drugs] and then just get bored or just give up. . . . It doesn't make any sense. I just decide to do it." In contrast to the white women, nearly all of the black women became involved with drugs "because it was everywhere." Mary began smoking crack in her late twenties because "it was always around in those days." (She stopped using shortly after we met her when, after many years of waiting, she received stable housing in a calm and well-maintained building for senior citizens.) Vanessa, a black woman who describes herself as "slow" both in terms of her abilities when she was in school and her social life, started using crack at age thirty-seven, "because I was trying to follow everyone else, be like everyone else." Now in her forties, she wants to stop using ("I'm tired"), but finds that living in what she calls a "drug-infested neighborhood" makes it hard to step away from crack. For black women far more than for white women, subpar schools, racially discriminatory hiring practices, and segregated and impoverished neighborhoods present insurmountable challenges to building the kinds of lives they wish for. As Tonya, a black woman who happens to be one of Anasia's former drug dealers explains, "As soon as you [a potential employer] see me, you don't think 'maybe she has skills.' They just have stereotypes—'ghetto black.'"

RACIAL SEGREGATION AND MASS INCARCERATION

Anasia, like many other women of color, grew up in a segregated community that had been systematically excluded from the economic and social opportunities of the late twentieth and early twenty-first centuries (Lipsitz 2012). Throughout the last decades of the twentieth century and into the twenty-first, deindustrialization—the closing down of manufacturing jobs—has disproportionately impacted African Americans (Costa Vargas 2006). By the second decade of the new millennium one-quarter of African Americans lived on incomes below the federal poverty level (FPL, which in 2013 was an annual income of $11,490 for a single person and $23,550 for a family of four). This rate is twice that of white Americans living below the FPL (Macartney, Bishaw, & Fontenot 2013). Nationally, black women experience higher poverty rates than either white women or black men (Ezeala-Harrison 2010).

Historian George Lipsitz (2012) draws particular attention to the deleterious effects of race-based housing segregation. White flight to the suburbs, lax or nonexistent enforcement of fair housing laws, redlining, predatory lending, exclusionary zoning, real estate steering, and refusing to rent or sell to members of targeted groups, all produce and intensify racially segregated housing patterns.[2] Housing segregation promotes the concentration of poverty in neighborhoods inhabited largely by blacks and Latinos. Concentrations of poverty, in turn, propel inequalities in resources and services. Poor minority neighborhoods are characterized by underfunded schools, inadequate health care services, lack of reasonably priced nutritious food, overcrowding, air and noise pollution from factories and mass transit hubs, and crumbling buildings (Williams and Mohammed 2009; Osypuk and Acevedo-Garcia 2010). Rates of lead poisoning are higher in poor and black neighborhoods (Bullard 1994); in New York, a black child is 8.5 times more likely than a white child to be exposed to lead poisoning (Hanley 2008). Recent statistical research shows that while black youth continue to be arrested at rates substantially higher than those of their white peers, crime rates among black youth began to fall vis-à-vis white youth when, in the wake of removal of lead from gasoline in 1988–1991, the difference in rates of elevated lead levels fell from six times higher for black children to "only" three times higher (Nevin 2013).

By the time Anasia was a teenager, both unemployment and the crack epidemic had begun to sweep through inner-city neighborhoods, and her two older brothers were incarcerated for drug involvement. "Crack was a marketing innovation" of the mid-1980s (Reinarman and Levine 1997). Powder cocaine, which had been around for decades, was expensive. But processed into the more powerful smokable form of crack cocaine, the drug could be sold on the street in small quantities to residents of impoverished inner-city neighborhoods. This marketing innovation succeeded, in part because of the availability of a huge workforce of unemployed young people ready to take jobs in the new, neighborhood-based business of crack preparation and sales (Reinarman and Levine 1997). This was an unemployed workforce that, as discussed in chapter 2, had been created by neoliberal "trickle down" policies, incentives to move factories overseas, and disinvestment from working-class communities.

Although the so-called War on Drugs was launched well before the crack cocaine innovation (see chapter 7), it has resulted in unprecedented rates of imprisonment in black communities. George Lipsitz argues that mandatory sentencing, harsher sentences for crack cocaine than for powder cocaine possession, more severe penalties for minor crimes, and "stop and frisk" policies "emerged as part of a counterrevolution against the democratic and egalitarian reforms of the mid-twentieth century that made more rights available to more people—as a result of the civil rights movement. This counterrevolution has used moral panics about crime as an ideological tool to reduce the number of rights-bearing citizens, to stigmatize members of aggrieved social groups, and to prevent workers from bargaining freely over wages and working conditions by rendering them displaceable, disposable, and deportable" (Lipsitz 2012). Mass incarceration is thus "linked to goals of maintaining inequality, scapegoating marginalized groups, and promoting economic benefit for social, political, and corporal elites" (Richie 2012, p. 21).

In the propaganda of the War on Drugs, the human face of both the victims and the dealers are disproportionately black or brown. Judith Scully (2002) traces public comments made by President George H. W. Bush, a central figure during a key period of the War on Drugs, in which he declared—and journalists reiterated—that the drug problem in America is most severe in public housing projects (a euphemism for the black community). Bush's own drug policy director, William J. Bennett, acknowledged that this was not the case; that the typical drug user is a white male who graduated from high school, is employed, and does not live in the inner city. "Consistent with this philosophy," however, Scully notes, "the nation's war on drugs has focused almost exclusively on low-level dealers and users in African-American neighborhoods. Police find drugs in these communities because that is where they look for them. Had they pointed the war at college campuses, it is likely that American jails would now be filled overwhelmingly with white university students who are both using and selling drugs" (2002, p. 59).

Black Americans are far more likely than white Americans to be incarcerated. Nationally, in December 2012, 463 out of every 100,00 white men; 2,841 out of every 100,000 black men; and 1,158 out of every 100,000 Hispanic men were incarcerated. The numbers for women, while smaller, reflect the same racial profile: .49 per 100,000 white women; 115 per 100,000 black women; and 64 per 100,000 Hispanic women are incarcerated (Carson & Golinelli 2013). Racial inequalities within the correctional system start early. African American girls are less likely to be diverted from the criminal system into educational or therapeutic programs; they receive the least amount of lenient treatment for offenses; and they are half as likely as female white youth to have the charges against them dismissed (American Bar Association & National Bar Association 2001).[3]

ANASIA

Once Anasia had finished the program at the halfway house where she had been living when we first met her, she moved into what is called a sober house (in this case, overpriced rooms rented to "recovering addicts"). For Anasia, a woman who prided herself on her neatly cut short hair, nicely pressed jeans, and well-groomed appearance, the sober house was "chaos." It was actually more of a "crack house." Anasia explained: "[I] just lived there and got high. It is a disgusting place. You never know if a bullet is going to come through the wall. It is one street away from last week's murders. I was on that street earlier in the evening. Now I just make sure I go to the next street. All that goes on there is drug stuff. People get real touchy when you are messing with their money and there is a lot of money to be made." After the crack house, "I was staying at my sisters for a while, but she was shooting drugs, and I had to get away from all that. It's a mess."

Without access to a decent education or to social networks of people working in good jobs, Anasia's employment options were limited. Throughout her adult life, Anasia moved between shoplifting and prostitution, and legal jobs in stores and nursing homes. A few years after we first met her, a white friend helped her get a job as a home health aide for a physically disabled woman who needed a great deal of lifting. The job paid $11.60 an hour, with no benefits. Anasia quit the job when her employer called her "nigger." We have never seen Anasia as angry as she was the day she told us about this. "If she did not like the way I was working, that would be one thing. No one calls me a nigger." The woman apologized and asked her to come back, but Anasia had no interest in "wiping the behind" of an overt racist.

A year or so after the home health aide incident, she worked at a department store until she was caught stealing. But in truth, Anasia confided, she would not have lasted much longer in the job anyway. With arthritis in both hips and both knees, she has trouble walking and standing. "Arthritis from too many burglaries, too much running from the police, too much jumping out windows, and too much drug use." Doctors have told her she needs to have surgery, but she can't afford not to work, so she keeps delaying the surgery. In the meantime, any legal jobs she can get involve lifting heavy people or boxes, exacerbating her health challenges. Nonlegal sources of income, of course, increase her risk of being arrested; each arrest adds to her criminal record, further constraining her job options and further locking her into the caste of the ill and afflicted.

Racist attitudes and practices take a toll. Nationally, among blacks, infant mortality rates are higher and adult life expectancy is lower than for whites at all levels of income and education. Death rates among African Americans are higher than among white Americans for most of the fifteen leading causes of death; this disparity has persisted over time, and in some aspects (most notably infant mortality) has widened (Williams & Mohammed 2009; CDC 2011; MacDorman & Mathews 2011). Blacks are also more likely than whites to live with chronic pain (Massoglia 2008b). Anasia's experience as a home health aide to a racist client helps explain these disparities. Not only are her hips, knees, and back worn down by years of lifting heavy patients, but her sense of being in the world is worn down by the insults, fears, indignities, and worries of living with racism. For Anasia, as for millions of Americans, both the material conditions of poverty and the stress of persistent discrimination damage the cardiovascular and immune systems, weakening the body's ability to fight off disease and sometimes leading to unhealthy behaviors such as smoking in order to manage the pain and stress (Braveman et al. 2010; Olshansky et al. 2012; Pascoe & Richman 2009; Williams & Mohammed 2009). Given the disproportionate rates of incarcerating Americans of color, it is worth emphasizing that the health status of blacks relative to whites has worsened during the period of mass incarceration (Sabol 2011).

INTERSECTIONS OF RACE AND GENDER, PART 2

Throughout American history black women's bodies—and especially their sexuality—have been targeted for control, exploitation, and assault. Under slavery white men literally owned black women's bodies; a slave woman's children did not belong to her, and rape of a black slave by a white "owner" was not considered a crime. To the contrary, it was an integral component of the master-slave relationship both in terms of producing more slaves to work the land and in terms of enforcing gender and racial hierarchies (Roberts 1997). In the twentieth-century, myths about black women's hypersexuality were used to justify involuntary sterilization and medical experimentation (Roberts 1997). As we discuss in chapter 2, late-twentieth-century and early-twenty-first-century welfare policy as articulated in the Personal Responsibility and Work Opportunity Act institutionalizes thinly disguised ideas that poor and black women do not control their fertility properly and so need to be regulated via policies such family caps on welfare eligibility. By the end of the twentieth century the myth of "crack babies" born to irresponsible black mothers ("crack whores") captured the American imagination and was driven by media reports predicting that the United States would shortly face an unprecedented crisis of babies who, due to prenatal cocaine exposure, would be born with terrible cognitive impairments that would require lifelong support from the state. The feared "crack babies" never materialized; studies show that use of crack by pregnant women actually did not give rise to predicted developmental and other disabilities in the infants born to these women (Hallam Hurt, cited in FitzGerald 2013). Yet these ideas continue to drive public beliefs and policies.

Except during the height of the "crack baby" moral panic, greater attention has been given to the mass incarceration of black men than of black women, both within the black community and in the white-dominated media. While black men are portrayed as "gangstas" and "gangbangers," black women are cast as "welfare queens." In reality, the white women of our project tended to use far more social services than did the black women. Still, we occasionally heard a white woman make thinly veiled racist comments about "those people" who "cheat the system and collect welfare and drive Cadillacs." Though derogatory (implying welfare fraud and low-level criminality), the term *welfare queen* also suggests that the state helps black women and even that it has generously stepped in and filled the shoes of black husbands and fathers who are too unreliable to care for their own families. Casting the state as savior of black women, of course, obscures the reality that in urban black neighborhoods affected by mass incarceration, large numbers of men exit prison to find that their criminal records bar them from ever obtaining employment in the legal economy and that they are permanently unable to afford stable housing or to support their families.

As Lipsitz explains (2012, p. 68), "Black women and Latinas endure injustices on their own, but they also suffer from the neighborhood race effects and collateral consequences of the mass incarceration of black and Latino men." Mass incarceration disrupts gender balances in ways that may allow the smaller number of men remaining in the community to exert greater power in their relationships with women, including the power to demand multiple sexual partners (Thomas & Torrone, 2006).[4] The consequences for black women are multifaceted. Drawn into what Beth Richie (2012, p. 36) calls the "trap of loyalty," black women live with the obligation to buffer their families from the impact of racism in the public sphere; pressure to live up to expectations that they as black women will better withstand abuse and mistreatment than other people; and acceptance of community rhetoric that claims that black women are in a more privileged position than black men.

Anasia's experiences with men during the years we have known her attest to these challenges. One day, over a cheeseburger and Pepsi, she told us that she had started going out with Jack. "He is a really nice guy," she said. "He is a Reverend! He used drugs when he was younger, then went to prison for a long time. He is very smart, and went to school and everything. He has been drug free a long time." Anasia continued to sing Jack's praises for another year or so. Then, over another cheeseburger and Pepsi, she announced that she was done with Jack. "He was screwing around. I don't need that." For a few months Anasia did not hear from Jack. And then she reported, "Jack just got out of jail. I don't know what he was in for. I want nothing to do with him. It was all lies anyway. I am done with him. He called yesterday, and I told him I was done with him. He didn't seem to believe it."

A year or so later Anasia became involved with another man. Before long she let us know, "My new boyfriend is in the hospital. He was beaten up and has broken ribs and cuts on his head. I sure can pick 'em, can't I? He drinks and gets drunk and picked a fight with a guy. He won that one, but then some of the guy's friends jumped him and beat him up. Now his family wants to come and get the guys who beat him up." This feud put Anasia in danger. Black women, in particular, suffer from assaults that are extensions of hostility between men (Richie 2012, p. 38).

In her own way, Anasia has explained to us that immersion of large numbers of black men in hypermasculine prison environments exacerbates sexual violence both inside and outside of prison. Indeed, studies show that communities with high rates of unemployed, insecurely housed, and formerly incarcerated residents tend to suffer high rates of street violence, increasing the chances that women and girls will be sexually assaulted (Coker et al. 2011). Beth Richie (2012, esp. p. 43) documents particularly high rates of sexual violence, including remarkably brutal forms of violence (multiple perpetrators, use of weapons or objects) carried out against black women by black men. And data indicate that while mandatory arrest policies for domestic violence may sometimes serve as a deterrent for men who feel that they have something to lose by being incarcerated, men with little to lose, socially and economically, often become more violent in response to arrest (Mills 2003). Coming full circle, black women are disproportionately likely to be evicted from their housing by landlords in the wake of calling the police to intervene in situations of domestic violence (Desmond & Valdez 2012).

Four years after first meeting Anasia, we asked her how she feels her life has been affected by her childhood experiences of racism in the Boston housing projects.

Yes, there was a lot of people who hated blacks and would pick on me, but I don't think being black was what made a difference in my life. There is a lot of racism, and not all blacks end up like me. I made my own choices—bad choices—but they were my own. Yes, I guess some of the schools that I went to until I quit could have been better, but again, not everyone that went to that school ended up in prison. I just made my own path. What is interesting is that my best friends have almost always been white. Even in the housing project, my best friend was white. Even now my best friend is white. I don't really see them as white, but as who they are. I guess I do have some prejudices, like against Puerto Ricans. Where my mom lives is now all Puerto Rican. Since they have moved in, the place has really gone downhill.

There is still a lot of racism, but you just deal with it, you live with it. Like when Obama was inaugurated, only the black women [in the rehabilitation facility where we first met her] watched it on the TV. One of the other black women saw that all the white women in the house had left the room. Later one of the white women said, "Hey, we should have something for St Patrick's Day," and I thought they sure didn't make a suggestion for Martin Luther King Day. It is there and it's everywhere, but you just keep on . . . you notice, but what are you going to do? If I had said anything about MLK, that woman would not have understood. . . . I don't think the police are racist. . . . At least with me. There are probably some who are. But they know me very well. All the police in town know me. I did the crime and I got caught. When they arrest me, they know me. The last time they simply said, "It is time to come in, Anasia," and I knew. It wasn't like they were targeting me but more like they knew I was playing fast and loose way too often, and it was time for me to stop it. The same with the courts. They have given me many, many chances. I once stayed clean for over two years and then used again, and then they give me another chance.

Whether Anasia truly believes what she told us about race or whether she told us what she believed we wanted to hear,[5] it is clear that she is well versed in the popular American script that attributes suffering to one's own bad choices and character defects. Even when acknowledging that racism is "everywhere," the example she offers has to do with the ignorance of a couple of homeless, marginalized white women regarding a particular individual—Martin Luther King, Jr. The police, in contrast, she described as not racially biased—a description that begs explanation in light of well-known practices of racial profiling and the obvious overrepresentation of black men and women in jails and prisons.

For the women in this project, gender typically seems to trump race. Race is not institutionally labeled in the way that gender is. Prisons, homeless shelters, and rehabilitation programs are not officially racially segregated, but they are officially gender segregated. Being a victim of gendered violence is a recognized status both in the correctional system and in the social welfare and therapeutic systems; being a victim of racism is not. Gendered explanations for women's misery are preached and drilled in the many facilities and programs in which women serve time. Racial explanations, if mentioned at all, are likely dismissed as "playing the race card."

Like Anasia, few of the project women—black or white—make much reference to race or racism. Melanie, a white woman who has been both a longtime client and, recently, a caseworker on the institutional circuit, mused that in her experience, "in the system, race doesn't really matter. What matters is shady cops who make women do things [have sex] with them or they turn them in." Perhaps, as Michelle Alexander (2012) points out, the supposed race neutrality of the War on Drugs makes it hard for society to see the racism that drives disparities in rates of arrest and punishment. Perhaps we Americans want to believe that racism (like other attitudes underlying hate crimes) denotes individual "bad" behavior rather than policies and attitudes that are core aspects of our history and social structure. Because racism is deeply embedded in American culture, it persists in institutions even when individuals do not profess racist attitudes (Williams & Mohammed 2009). Perhaps people such as Anasia and Melanie grow up in circumstances in which racism is so much a part of the air they breathe that they come to take it for granted, and it becomes hard to see as a distinct and nameable phenomenon.

Tonya, who was raised in a middle-class black family, is the only project participant who consistently offered race-based observations and interpretations. When we asked her why, in her opinion, other women seem tuned out to racism, she mulled the question over and replied that men's prisons are very racially divided but women's prisons are not. After giving examples of the race-based gangs and violence in men's prisons, Tonya explained that in women's prisons, "everyone is involved with everyone else, except for some of the Spanish-speaking women who keep to themselves." While racial tensions pop up from time to time, they rarely if ever resemble the overt racial hostility and violence that are characteristic of men's prisons. On another occasion we chatted with Tonya about race and mass incarceration. Her response echoed mainstream public discourse: black men are overincarcerated, not black women. While black men are seen as racial victims of mass incarcerations, the criminalization of black women tends to be ignored.

————

In real life, race and gender identities are never separate. Anasia is always both a black person and a woman, and the lived experiences of her blackness are gendered as much as her lived experiences as a woman are racialized. These two identities are mutually constitutive and structured in dominance.[6] The fact is that Anasia is more likely to be arrested and incarcerated than her white female counterparts, *and* she is more likely than her black male counterparts to be sexually assaulted and to be sent to so-called therapeutic programs in which she is taught that her problems lie within her own "victim mentality." Certainly at this point in her life Anasia feels that changing her own behavior seems more possible than changing racist beliefs, practices, and policies over which she has little control.

The neoliberal doctrine of personal responsibility that is drilled and drilled again in both correctional and therapeutic institutions serves to obscure racism and other structural causes of suffering from public consciousness. It seems to us that the valorization of personal responsibility in and of itself indexes culturally persistent racist images of dark-skinned people as "lazy" and "childlike" (Gilens 1999). Put differently, the language of personal responsibility has come to stand in for explicit references to race in an era in which we, as a society, would like to believe that we have put our history of racism behind us. Our cultural taboo on using the "N-word" or making explicitly racist comments does not mean that institutionalized racism has disappeared. To the contrary, in this age of mass incarceration, the structural manifestations of racism have escalated. As is disproportionately the case for black Americans, Anasia received a substandard education in a neighborhood with substandard apartment buildings housing a population that suffered from high rates of illness and incarceration. Because these systems feed and reinforce each other, there were few opportunities for Anasia to avoid a fate shaped by racism. Anasia couldn't catch a break, not because she dodged personal responsibility for making good choices, but because the systemic forces that constrain her choices are so very strong.

CHAPTER 4

Suffer the Women

Pain and Perfection in a Medicalized World

My using drugs—it was self-medication. And the drugs work!
—Donna

Touching her fingertips to her lips and blowing kisses around the room, Ginger made her rounds of the women's center, greeting friends and acquaintances with a steady stream of "Hello, Gorgeous!" and "Good Morning, Beautiful!" Tottering on high heels, she sighed aloud, "We girls have to suffer to be beautiful." She then got down to business sorting through the donated clothing in hopes of finding "something that will show off my ass." Although we had never spoken to her at length, we had seen Ginger at the women's center nearly every day. Sometimes she napped in an easy chair; sometimes she sashayed in and out, flashing her new wig or nails; but most often she helped the center's director wipe down tables, fold and sort donated clothing, pick up discarded candy wrappers from the floor, and clean out the coffee machine. On this particular day, Ginger made a beeline to the couch on which we were sitting and chatting with a few women. She had caught wind of our project and was eager to participate. We had to think quickly. Our goal was to understand the experiences of criminalized women, but Ginger had lived as a boy named George until she was sixteen years old. Still, how could we deny what we suspected was Ginger's earnest request that she, like the other women's center denizens, be validated as a woman?

A few months later Ginger disappeared from the scene, and no one seemed to know where she had gone. We looked for her at the Boston Common, where many homeless people hang out, and we tried calling a phone number she had given us a while back—it was disconnected. Assuming she was back in jail, we launched a campaign of calling friends who work in correctional facilities in order to find out to which jail we should go to visit her. None of our contacts could tell us anything. And then, a few weeks later, out of the blue, Ginger reappeared. "Where were you?" we asked. "Are you okay?" "Oh," Ginger replied, "my mother had hip replacement surgery, so I stayed with her at the hospital and then I went home with her because she needs help getting up." With only one other sibling (a brother), Ginger had taken on a role many daughters assume at some point in their lives: caring for an aging or infirm parent. That was the day we understood that we had not been humoring Ginger by "allowing" her to join our project.

———

Born into one of the working-class Irish neighborhoods involved in conflicts over Boston school desegregation in the 1970s, Ginger knew she was "not a regular boy" by age five or six when she dressed as a woman for Halloween and "didn't want to ever have to take off the costume." Her mother took her to doctors who told her, "It's a chromosome thing—extra female chromosomes, or maybe hormones." And for as long as she can remember, doctors have prescribed medication "to help me with my anger issues."

Like many children who are different from their peers, George was the target of abuse. When she was thirteen, her stepfather, who also beat her mother, molested her. When she was fourteen, she had sex with a man she had just met on a bus. Terrified that he may have infected her with AIDS, she swallowed a handful of pills, screamed, yelled, cut herself, and burned herself with cigarettes. Her mother committed her to a juvenile psychiatric hospital, where she was put in eight-point shackles, given a mood-stabilizing drug, and treated for PTSD.[1]

In the hospital she met a "queen" who lived in a working-class city north of Boston and invited Ginger to visit her there. "The queen showed me the ropes." "What ropes?" we asked. "Hustling." "When did you start using drugs?" we asked. "Where I grew up, lots of kids were using different drugs and I tried them out. But I didn't really use until after what happened on the bus." After a few more stints in hospitals and juvenile facilities, when she was fifteen, the psychiatrists who treated her signed the documentation certifying that she met Social Security's criteria for disability (SSI).[2] Ginger explains, "I've had therapists forever for bipolar and anger issues."

For the next year or so Ginger lived at home. In her neighborhood men were expected to be men and girls to be girls. Ginger recalls that her mother's house was repeatedly spray painted with the word *faggot*, rocks were thrown through the window, and her younger brother was forced to fight the other boys in the neighborhood on a regular basis. After a few particularly horrific attacks, Ginger left home in order to protect her family from further violence. Having heard that New York is the place to be "for girls like me," (Ginger's preferred term for transgender women) she headed there.

Young and petite, Ginger quickly found a job in a drag show, ingested female hormones "to grow titties," was introduced to crack, and earned money through sex work. Some transwomen experience prostitution (demonstrating female attractiveness to male clients) as affirming their female identity, but many trans/queer youth simply find their options for securing food and shelter limited to selling drugs, engaging in sex work, shoplifting, and scamming (Ware 2011). For Ginger both were true. She happily reminisces about working in the drag show and sharing an apartment with other "girls like me."

After a few years in New York, Ginger returned to Boston "because I wanted a husband who will love me for what I am. That's what a lot of girls want." Within a month of returning home, she met Clevon, the man she considers to be her husband. "He was my dealer and I was his 'ho,'" Ginger would tell anyone who will listen. More recently she clarified that each of them had his or her own "hustle" and that Clevon "was not a big-time dealer, just a straggler. He was never my pimp. But he always had my back." Although he clearly adores her, Clevon carries his own baggage. According to Ginger, "He is a little retarded; his brain is messed up. He was in foster care and lived on the streets since age ten." By age fifteen he was hustling, pimping, and using drugs. He has less than an elementary school education and cannot read or write. His criminal record makes him unemployable, and he is black, which in Boston means that he is stopped by the police on a regular basis.

Ginger, too, has been locked up on numerous occasions for drug possession and "common night walking" (one of her favorite expressions). Studies show that the proportion of transgender women who have a history of incarceration is as high as 67 percent, and that police and law enforcement officers are among the main perpetrators of acts of violence against lesbian, gay, bisexual, and transgender (LGBT) people (Mogul, Ritchie, & Whitlock 2011). According to a survey conducted in Washington, D.C., 16 percent of transgender respondents reported being sent to jail or prison for charges such as loitering, soliciting sex, possession of controlled substances, shoplifting, etc., with black (47%) and American Indian (30%) respondents at highest risk of going to jail or prison. Twenty-one percent of male-to-female transgender respondents reported having been sent to jail in contrast to 10 percent of female-to-male respondents (Xavier 2000). Nationally, transgender women are so frequently perceived to be sex workers by the police that the term *walking while trans* was coined as a derivative of the more commonly known *driving while black* (Mogul, Ritchie, & Whitlock 2011, p. 61).

Open and even chatty about almost all aspects of her life, Ginger does not talk about her experiences in men's prisons and has made it clear that we should not ask her about this period of her life. There is now a special carceral unit in Massachusetts for "girls like me," but when she was younger, Ginger was incarcerated as a man. Studies document horrifyingly high rates of violence against LGBT people in prison: more than half of LGBT inmates report having been sexually assaulted in prison—a rate fifteen times higher than that for the general prison population. In the hypermasculine cauldrons that are men's prisons, female transgenders are particularly likely to be targets of rape (Mogul, Ritchie, & Whitlock 2011), and gay and effeminate white men are especially targeted for punishment by white guards and prisoners for "making the white race weak" (Dillon 2011). Lacking access to appropriate medical treatment, some incarcerated transpeople injure themselves while trying to perform surgery on themselves or by sharing needles for hormone or silicone injections (Grant, Mottet, & Tanis 2011).

While Ginger prefers to talk about the positive people and events in her life, she acknowledges having been attacked and raped on the streets on many occasions. Sometimes the attackers were groups of drunken men who wanted to teach her a lesson. Others were boyfriends or sex-work clients who, denying that they are "queer" or "faggots," followed sex with a beating when they "suddenly realized that I'm not a girl." Her first boyfriend was abusive. "He threw me into a wall. He locked me in the apartment and yelled at me." Twenty years later, a few months after we met her, she was beaten up right outside the women's center by a former boyfriend who repeatedly punched her in the stomach.

Ginger has especially harsh words for pimps, explaining that girls hook up with pimps because they promise to take care of them and have their backs, but then they push the women to hustle more and more. When girls want to leave, the pimps don't let them, because they bring in $400 a night. She knows of pimps who followed girls to other cities to bring them back. We asked which comes first, crack or hustling. Ginger responded, "They come together. Girls use drugs to handle the hustling, but they also hustle to make money for drugs." Looking back on her life, though, Ginger muses, *"I got into that [sex work] to look for a husband, but I ended up with a crack habit."*

The consensus of the Boston women regarding street drugs is clear: drugs may be fun at first, but over the long run they will kill you. Ginger, like other women, has friends who were shot dead in front of her during drug deals that went bad, friends shot by law enforcement officers, and friends who died from overdoses. Virtually all of the project participants live with health problems related to drug use. More than half of the women have hepatitis C. Many have liver cirrhosis. Several have infections at injection points. Nearly three-quarters have overdosed or become deathly ill from toxic substances mixed into street drugs at some point in their lives (cf. Chen & Lin 2009). And like Ginger, nearly all of the women have suffered sexual assault in the context of drug use. Melanie, the youngest project participant, recalled that when she began using drugs in her early teens, she was raped a number of times while passed out. "I didn't understand that this was rape—I mean, I know the sex had happened but didn't realize that it is considered rape. Maybe that is why I'm depressed and anxious," she told us, showing us the bottles of medication prescribed by her psychiatrist as "proof" (her word) that she "really" is sick.

DRUG LUST, PART I

On multiple levels, Ginger is a poster child for modern medicine—for its attempt to solve socially induced and culturally construed suffering through drugs. Ginger was started on psychiatric medication when she was fifteen. According to Ginger, "Most people who use drugs have mental problems. In my case there is bipolar in my family but mostly what made my mental problems is society and people who can't accept me for what I am." Over the years she has been prescribed various mood stabilizers, including Depakote, but she generally does not take them. "They give them [to me] to numb me out, but that doesn't solve the problems," she tells us. She has taken female hormones (both prescribed and illicit)

TABLE I   PERCENTAGE OF ADULTS (18 YEARS AND OLDER)
WHO REPORTED USING ILLICIT SUBSTANCES, 2012

	Lifetime	Past year	Past month
Total	50.5	15.7	9.1
Gender			
Male	56.1	19.0	11.8
Female	45.3	12.7	6.6
Race			
White	54.1	15.7	9.2
Black	49.0	18.6	11.5
Hispanic	43.1	15.2	8.1
Education			
Less than high school	41.4	17.7	11.1
High school grad	48.8	15.8	9.8
College grad	51.6	12.4	6.6

SOURCE: SAMHSA 2013.

on and off for the past two decades. She also was a crack cocaine user for close to twenty years, and continues to smoke marijuana daily. Like most of the Boston women, Ginger typically interprets drug use as a response to miserable life circumstances, using the term "self-medicate" to explain why she uses drugs.[3]

In our highly medicalized society most of us look to drugs of one kind or another for "the key to a life free of illness, pain or suffering" (Crawford 2006, p. 404). According to a national survey by the Substance Abuse and Mental Health Services Administration (SAMHSA 2012), more than 23.9 million Americans aged twelve or older had used an illicit drug (such as cocaine, heroin, or methamphetamine) during the month prior to the survey interview. Over the past several years marijuana has been the most commonly used illicit drug, with illicit opiate use on the rise. In 2012, 4.9 million, or 1.9 percent, of the population made illicit use of prescription pain relievers (National Institute on Drug Abuse 2011). Approximately 15 percent of U.S. women and 30 percent of men drink alcohol at least three or four time a week (National Institute on Alcohol Abuse and Alcoholism 2014), and about 12 percent of American adults have had an alcohol dependence problem at some time in their life (Hasin et al. 2007). According to the 2012 National Survey on Drug Use and Health (SAMHS 2013), nearly a quarter of the population age twelve and older participated in what the study calls binge drinking (i.e., consuming five or more drinks during the same occasion) at least once in the past month; and more than 11 percent of the population drove under the influence of alcohol at least once in the year before the survey.

Legal use of prescription psychoactive and pain medications may be even more rampant. In 2010, 210 million (legal) prescriptions for opioids were written, a 276 percent increase from the 76 million prescriptions written in 1991. Prescriptions for stimulants rose in the same period from 4 million to 45 million (National Institute on Drug Abuse 2011). One in five adults currently takes a psychoactive medication. According to the U.S. Centers for Disease Control and Prevention (CDC 2011), more people are killed by prescription drugs than by illegal ones. In fact, prescription drug reactions and mistakes have become the nation's fourth leading cause of death.

The extent to which Americans use licit and illicit substances to numb physical or emotional pain or "normalize" feelings or behaviors, or to bring about some combination of these effects, prompts us to look beyond individualistic explanations for drug use (such as genetics or bad choices) and think about the broader social landscape in which so many people turn to drugs. Contented people who feel that their lives matter and are manageable may use mind-altering substances recreationally from time to time; that is the case throughout the world. But widespread chronic drug use, whether legal or illegal, must be seen as a consequence of social pathologies of various kinds.

Americans are becoming increasingly distressed. For example, a June 2013 Gallup poll revealed that 70 percent of Americans hate their jobs or have "checked out" of them (meaning they have become disengaged and do as little as possible; Sorenson & Garman 2013). While life may or may not be any more difficult than it was a generation ago, our belief in progress and our increased expectations that life should be ever more satisfying have resulted in mass disappointment. For many, society has become increasingly alienating, isolating, and downright mean. While in some instances social dissatisfaction fuels rebellion, in the United States today many feel hopeless about the possibility that political activism can create societal change. For those who have not given up hope in their own personal futures, Adderall and other medications used to treat ADHD (attention deficit/hyperactivity disorder) are often sold or passed around in suburban schools as a means to increase one's academic achievement and chances of future occupational and financial success (National Institute on Drug Abuse 2011). At the most empirical level, the 24/7 economy means that increasing numbers of Americans do shift and night work for which methamphetamine offers a useful way of staying awake.

———

Carl Hart is a neuroscientist who grew up in a poor, black urban neighborhood. Looking back at his own life experiences, he realized that he, like his peers, turned to crack in a period of economic decline in the inner cities when there were few other affordable sources of pleasure or purpose available to young people. However, when real choices were made available to him—initially, the chance to play basketball, a sport he excelled at, and later, the opportunity to join in anti-racism activism—he turned away from drugs.

Dissatisfied with broadly unquestioned assumptions regarding the nature of addiction, Hart has conducted experimental research in which drug users and addicts were offered a choice of crack or money. If the money incentive was more than a few dollars, but still less than the street value of the crack, many chose the money. "Basically, having choices makes an enormous difference," he explains, "even when drugs are involved. Cocaine isn't always the most compelling alternative, even for people whose lives seem to revolve around it. . . . The choice to use depends far more on context and availability of alternatives than we have been lead to believe" (Hart 2013, pp. 94–95).

Tonya, the opinionated woman introduced in chapter 3, has clear opinions about drug use: "It's not true that once an addict, always an addict [as they say in Narcotics Anonymous]. Someone fifteen years clean is not an addict [but in NA that is how they identify themselves]. The 1960s hippies [used drugs] and they moved on and are lawyers and teachers [not addicts]." In making this observation Tonya was arguing that if drug users have good choices—choices more appealing and meaningful than the high they get from drugs—they will make those good choices. To be clear, when talking about "choice," neither Hart nor Tonya is referring to the psychological choice to "get over" PTSD or develop self-esteem (see chapter 5), nor do they mean the pseudo-choice between homelessness and living with an abusive man (chapter 1) or the pointless "choice" to be economically self-sufficient when the only jobs available are part-time work at fast-food restaurants (chapter 2). Rather, both Hart and Tonya advocate for the sort of social and economic level playing field that allows all people—not just the elite few—a real chance at the American dream.

DRUG LUST, PART 2

Pharmaceutical companies have spent big advertising money over the past several decades to convince Americans that we are in some way deficient and that those deficiencies can best be addressed with drugs. On television, in magazines, and online, we as a nation are bombarded with advertisements telling us that we need drugs for high blood pressure, stress, erectile dysfunction, restless-leg syndrome, social anxiety disorder, hyperactivity, depression, asthma, hair loss, fatigue, loss of bladder control, menopause, and moodiness. Americans are now the most medicated people on the planet, and the pharmaceutical industry spends more money on advertising than on research. According to the Centers for Disease Control and Prevention (Qiuping, Dillon, & Burt 2010) in the month prior to its survey, 48 percent of Americans took at least one prescription drug. In 2008, $234.1 billion was spent in the United States on prescription drugs—more than double what was spent in 1999. In 2010, Americans spent $16 billion on legal antipsychotics, $11 billion on antidepressants, and $7 billion on drugs to treat ADHD (Smith 2012).

From Big Pharma's perspective, the Boston women have been good consumers. Like Ginger, Francesca (introduced in chapter 1) has been on psychiatric medication since age thirteen, in the wake of the abuse she endured as a child. In her mid-twenties, beaten up by her husband, she became addicted to Percocet. When we first met her, she was supposed to be taking "Seroquel plus Ativan [anti-anxiety medication] as needed," but had decided not to take it, because "I was tired of all the meds that made me a zombie—Prozac and the other meds." A year or so later she returned to her doctor and was put on Klonopin (anti-anxiety medication), Neurontin, Abilify, Ritalin (for ADD), and Trazodone (an antidepressant and anti-anxiety medication). She typically sells the Klonopin to buy Percocet. While there is little scientific information concerning the interactions among this cocktail of mood-altering substances, Francesca can vouch for the fact that quickly adding another prescription after the last often leaves her less capable of managing her already chaotic life (Chadwick, Waller, & Edwards 2005).

Elizabeth, whom we introduced in chapter 2, routinely falls asleep on an easy chair in the noisy women's center or on a blanket in the Boston Common. Shortly after we first met her, she told us that her grogginess was instigated by a new medication, Lamictal (an anticonvulsant used to treat bipolar disorder), which was causing her to have trouble concentrating and her speech to be slurred. She was especially concerned about the grogginess because in the past her belongings had been stolen while she napped outside. A year or so later her doctor added Celexa and Trazodone to her regimen. About a year after that, she was given Klonopin (which was stolen). A few months later she was back in prison, where she was put on Thorazine and Lithium (medications typically used for psychosis, though to the best of our knowledge, Elizabeth has never been diagnosed with any type of psychosis, nor do we see any behaviors that suggest psychosis). "This made me gain weight and made me into a space shot. It's not the right medicine. I'm not crazy; that's for crazy people. I have PTSD and depression. I refused to take the medicine. Then they put me on Prozac, but it didn't help." Since leaving prison, she has been put on Wellbutrin, Lamictal, and Ambien (the last, insomnia medication).

While some psychiatric medications for some people may be effective over the short term, these drugs may increase the likelihood that a person will become chronically ill over the long term (Kirk, Gomory, & Cohen 2013). Large-scale studies by the National Institute of Mental Health and the World Health Organization show little evidence that antipsychotics improve long-term schizophrenia outcomes; to the contrary, they may worsen long-term outcomes, and long-term recovery rates are higher for people who are not medicated (Kirk, Gomory, & Cohen 2013, pp. 118ff.). Similarly, there is compelling evidence that use of antidepressants actually increases depressive episodes in the long term; that as use of antidepressants increases, the number of Americans who report being depressed increases; and certain antidepressants have been linked to increased risk of suicide. Of particular concern for the Boston women, many of whom have been diagnosed with bipolar disorder, is evidence that sustained use of bipolar medication may result in long-term cognitive deficits and emotional numbing. Studies suggest that prolonged use of psychiatric medications may not only worsen target symptoms over the long run by permanently impacting neurotransmitter pathways, but also seems to be associated with a range of physical problems, including metabolic illnesses, kidney failure, and cardiovascular ailments (Whitaker 2010, p. 211).

The women of our project most often say that they use drugs to "numb" their emotional and physical pain. It is clear to us that drug use restricts their creativity in responding to and making meaning out of suffering. While illicit drugs most directly constrain autonomy when women fall into the power webs of dealers and the correctional system, legally prescribed psychotropic drugs also must be seen as constraining autonomy, especially those drugs designed to help with "impulse control" or "anger issues." or those prescribed as a requirement for regaining housing or custody of one's children.[4]

THE WAR ON DRUG (USERS)

The majority of the Boston women began their psychiatric medication, as well as their street drug careers, as teenagers. Like Ginger, nearly all of the women continued to use both—sequentially or concurrently—as adults. We have learned that it is not always useful to make sharp distinctions between legal and illegal drugs. Both may be used for the same reasons (to "feel better"), and both impact the brain at the neuronal level; methamphetamine and Adderall, for instance, are essentially the same drug (Hart 2013). Further blurring the distinctions, psychiatric medications are widely used to treat addiction to illegal drugs; alcoholics are often treated with antidepressants such as valium and other benzodiazepines in the early withdrawal phase; and methadone, a highly addictive synthetic opioid, is widely used to treat heroin addiction.

Barbara Herbert, chief of addiction services at St. Elizabeth Medical Center in Brighton, Massachusetts (near Boston), attributes the overuse of pain medication, in part, to insurance companies' willingness to pay for relatively inexpensive prescription pain medication rather than for extensive physical therapy, acupuncture, or other nonpharmacological interventions. "I see a number of people who come through our program who have slid from using medication because of an injury or because of a good, real reason, to using it because it gives them the energy to do their housework or lets them finish working extra hours at their jobs, to not being able to afford it anymore, to using heroin" (Herbert, quoted in Chapman 2013; cf. Canfield 2010).

Although the distinction between licit and illicit drug use may look like a choice, the use of one or the other is often a function of what a person can get ahold of. For many low-income Americans, especially those without health insurance, legal psychotropic or pain medication is hard to come by. Affluent Americans with good health insurance may find it almost too easy to receive prescriptions for psychotropic medication. Ginger, like many of the Boston women, experiences severe anxiety and panic attacks for which her "drug of choice" is Klonopin (one of a class of drugs called benzos [benzodiazepines] that include Xanax, Ativan, and Valium). While an informal survey of Susan's friends indicates that middle-class women are likely to be offered these drugs by their doctors for help with issues ranging from menopause to long airplane flights, incarcerated women in Massachusetts are not given benzodiazepines as a matter of policy (even if they were taking them per a doctor's prescription at the time they entered prison) because of concern that benzos are addictive and, as we were told by several correctional officers, that women will sell or trade them.

———

The legal status of particular substances has changed over time. A century ago, heroin and cocaine were legal, nonprescription drugs. During prohibition, alcohol sales were illegal. And after decades of locking up Americans on marijuana charges, marijuana has been decriminalized in a number of states and legalized in a few other states. As a society we tend to divide and polarize drugs, seeing certain ones as evil and other, quite similar (or even identical) ones as life-saving pinnacles of American scientific and medical progress. During the same decades when spending on and use of prescription psychotropic medication proliferated, street drugs became the focus of a full-blown moral panic—the so-called War on Drugs. Looking at the foundational rhetoric of the War on Drugs, James Hawdon (2001) traced the way Ronald Reagan and Nancy Reagan consistently framed drug use as a conscious choice, with the implication that it is appropriate to punish drug users (because they could have said no to drugs.) "In this way social problems [are] construed as the moral failings of the individual" (Hawdon 2001, p. 428). Indeed, the United States has a long history of public crusades to stamp out personal vices and diseases (the two words often are used interchangeably), ranging from masturbation and homosexuality to alcohol use and obesity (cf. Szasz 1992).

From the start, the War on Drugs did not rely on systematic evidence for its justification, but rather played on cultural fears. In fact, at the time the War on Drugs was declared in 1971, drug use was actually declining. The timing is significant. The launch of the drug war coincided with the peak of social movements for racial equality. By targeting black communities, the War on Drugs functioned, intentionally or not, to defuse the threat that the civil rights movement posed to the racially hierarchical status quo (Alexander 2012).

The War on Drugs rapidly slipped into a War on Drug Users, the central weapon of which has been mass incarceration of poor Americans of color (Wacquant 2009; Garland 2001; Haney 2010).[5] Nationally, incarceration rates skyrocketed between 1980 and 1993, from 130 to 322 per 100,000 people; drug-related charges accounted for the lion's share of that growth. It is no coincidence that this is the same period during which economic policies created widening gaps between rich and poor (see chapter 2) and during which disinvestment from low-income communities became "accepted as an inevitable consequence of individual pathology" (Richie 2012, p. 113).

The War on Drugs is big business, fueling what has come to be called the "prison industrial complex" (Sudbury 2005). Current spending to fund the Drug War, which includes police, courts, and prisons, is estimated at over $40 billion a year (G. Becker & Murphy 2013), and since its onset in 1971 the United States has spent an estimated $1 trillion on the war (Branson 2012). Yet with all of this money poured into what is becoming the longest "war" in American history, the amount of illicit drugs available globally has steadily increased. The Global Commission on Drug Policy (2011, p. 2) recently declared, "The global war on drugs has failed, with devastating consequences for individuals and societies around the world (see also UNODC 2011, p. 1). According to Helen Clark, head of the United Nations Development Program, "There is increasing evidence that the war on drugs has failed with criminalization often creating more problems than it solves" (Stargardter 2013).

GINGER

When we first met Ginger, she was in her thirties and had pretty much stopped working as a prostitute. "I'm tired of it—the crack, waking in the morning not knowing if I have money for a cigarette, coffee. It costs a lot for a girl to look beautiful at my age—cosmetics, all that." Ginger explained that as she got older, her body changed, it became harder for her to stay slim, and the customers "want new faces." She would dye her hair to look different, and that would work for a bit, but then customers would realize it was her. She found it increasingly difficult to stand around all night trying to attract a few men. At a local ladies' bingo night, where Ginger and her cousin have long been enthusiastic players (Ginger informally serves as hostess, cheerleader, and comic relief), she even showed up once or twice with a five o'clock shadow. In the time we have known her, she has trended away from dressing in drag, often saying she is "too tired" to put the effort into "being a girl."

Feeling that Boston had become a trap for her—too many people knew her and tempted her with crack and a lifestyle she no longer wanted—a few years after we first met, Ginger decided to move to Florida to live with her brother, his wife, and their baby. Working hard at building up a business, her brother and his girlfriend were thrilled that Ginger would be able to look after the child. For the first few months in Florida, things went swimmingly (literally—she loved the beach). When we chatted on the phone, she told us that she had even landed a part-time job promoting a drag club on Sunday evenings. She was paid to stand outside the door for several hours and persuade customers to come in. "I love it. I get to dress as a girl and people here love seeing me and like to take their pictures with me. There aren't many trannies around here and people love me."

But, as Francesca found when the thrill of a new place began to wear off, the structural obstacles that made Ginger's life difficult in Boston were the same, or worse, in Florida. The drag club paid her under the table and only wanted her twice a week for four hours a shift. That did not provide enough money for her to pay rent for her own apartment after her relationship with her brother's wife deteriorated. During one phone call with us Ginger was in tears because the wife had berated her for spending $50 on boots rather than saving the money to get an apartment. Ginger explained to us that the problem was that rents were very high in Florida and public transportation minimal, so she was limited in terms of finding another place. Also, she hadn't been able to make friends in Florida and found that, aside from the job at the club, she was not safe going out in public dressed as Ginger rather than as George. "There is nothing to do here, nowhere to go, no friends; everything is expensive. I don't want to leave my nephew, but my sister-in-law is twenty-six and she disrespects me. I'm thirty-nine. It's chaos, chaos. I'm living on an island and I'm suffocating. I'm from Boston and that's it. I'll never be a Florida local."

After less than a year she returned to Boston. Back home, she complained, "I'm tired, I don't want to live like that anymore." The next few times we ran into her, Ginger was dressed in jeans and a flannel shirt or in a tracksuit. She no longer kept her face free of hair, and she rarely wore makeup. We had just about become accustomed to the "new" Ginger when she stopped by the women's center to announce that she had just seen a doctor and would be starting a course of female hormones. Bursting with excitement, she told us that she was especially looking forward to having hormonal mood swings like other women. "I'm gonna yell at my husband. And I'm gonna tell him I have a headache when he wants sex," she exclaimed. A few weeks later she came by our office to tell us that her doctor had put her on Depakote, a mood stabilizer; Spiritactone, female estrogen; and Spiral, hormones. She was thrilled. "I'm getting hot flashes and mood swings like a real woman!"

GENDERING DRUGS: HORMONES AND COSMETIC SURGERY

The many ups and downs we have heard about and have witnessed throughout our relationship with Ginger puts into focus both the power of oppressive gender social norms to cause suffering and the ways in which medicalization and criminalization work in tandem to sustain gender norms and correct or punish those who transgress those norms. Ginger ran away from home because she was beaten up for being a "faggot," took to the street as a prostitute, and was thrown into a men's jail where, as a "queen," she endured unspeakable violence. Over the same years, Ginger made ample use of prescribed and illicit psychotropic drugs in order to cope with the violence she experienced, and she dabbled in another sort of drug—female hormones—to bring her outward appearance in line with social expectations for how women *should* look.

Like "regular women" (her words), Ginger spends a great deal of time and money on cosmetics, hair removal, and hair extensions. And like many American women, Ginger utilizes modern medicine in her efforts to perform gender: to correct what she perceives as wrong in her body and face so that men will find her desirable. The hormones that help Ginger align her sense of self with her outward appearance are the same hormones millions of middle-aged women have been prescribed for much the same reason. Indeed, hormone replacement therapy has been marketed as a means for women to maintain a youthful and feminine appearance when their outward appearance no longer fits social norms for feminine beauty and desirability. Many of Ginger's friends also have sought the same cosmetic surgeries undergone by millions of "regular" American women. She expresses a mixture of disdain and envy for "girls like me who have a sugar daddy" who will pay for breast implants, butt enhancements, facial feminization surgery (brow lift, rhinoplasty, cheek implantation, lip augmentation, Adam's apple reduction, jaw recontouring, and collagen injections), and hair transplants. These body-changing procedures involve significant medical risks, including pain, bleeding, and infection yet have become standard components of the American cosmetic-medical repertoire.

GINGER

Throughout her twenties and thirties, Ginger maintained her relationship with Clevon. "We were made for each other," she told us. While her mother would jest that "[they] are a match made in hell," Clevon was accepted into the family fold. They like him, Ginger said, because "he doesn't beat me and he still loves me." He and Ginger have ups and downs, breakups, and reconciliations. "I can't live with him and can't live without him."

Ginger feels blessed to have a supportive family. She is close not only to her brother but to a large number of cousins, aunts, nieces, and nephews. But the most important person in her life is her mother. She knows that her mother is always there for her, and she often declared that this bond is special because "she carried me in her stomach for nine months so there will never be anyone who is as close to me as my mother." They speak on a daily basis. When they each receive their respective monthly disability checks, they go out shopping together for a "mother-daughter" day. When we asked Ginger whether her mother treats her like a daughter or a son, she replied, "It depends on her mood. When she's in a good mood it's 'Ginger.' When she's in a bad mood it's 'George.' When she's in the middle it's 'G.'"

But not everything in her family life ran smoothly. Four years or so into our relationship, Ginger called to say that her mother had been rushed to the hospital. At first the doctors thought she had a brain tumor; as it turned out, she did not, but Ginger spent two weeks at her bedside helping her mother cope physically and emotionally. When her mother was released from the hospital, she was told that she would need a great deal of help at home; the doctor recommended that the family arrange for Ginger to be hired as a home health aide. But a few days later we ran into her hanging out in the Boston Common, so upset that she was trembling and barely able to talk. Her mother's husband (they have been married for about a decade; Ginger's own father is deceased) had accused Clevon of "touching" his grandson. He then began screaming at Ginger about her bringing "niggers" into the house. She was furious and threw a table and broke it. She is sure that Clevon did not do this; her mother's husband had previously accused Clevon's friend of the same thing. (Indeed, he later acknowledged that Clevon never molested the child.) Ginger told us that she would like to really hurt her mother's husband, "beat him in the head with a baseball bat." The upshot was that she was barred from the house and could not take care of her mother. Although this happened in September, Ginger spoke repeatedly about the holidays, saying she wouldn't be able to go to her mother's house for Christmas and would have to meet her mother at Dunkin Donuts to exchange gifts. A few weeks later things were patched up enough for Ginger to be able to go to her mother's house when the husband was out, but she has not forgotten the homophobic and racist poison he spewed, and she expressed worry that the next time something like this happens, "I'm going to totally lose it and end up in jail."

We caught a glimpse of the way Ginger and Clevon manage their relationship when we went to court with Ginger for her final "wrap"—a happy occasion when the judge officially informed her that she had completed parole and had no outstanding warrants. Clevon came to court but did not walk with her into the courtroom. Ginger, dressed as a boy, sat with Susan on a bench with a dozen or so white men and women. Clevon walked to a bench toward the back where several other black men were sitting. Ginger and Clevon did not speak to one another until we were a block or so away from the courthouse. When Susan offered to buy iced coffees to celebrate, Ginger and Clevon exchanged glances—the kind of unspoken communication common between longtime couples—asking whether Clevon should come inside the coffee shop and sit with us, or whether it would be better for him to drink his coffee outside. We later asked Ginger what this was about since we had often seen them together at the Boston Common. "I wasn't looking for trouble," Ginger explained.

———

As of this writing, Ginger is still insecurely housed, poor, and vulnerable to assault. However, she is one of the few Boston women to have consistently described herself as happy. She tells us that she stopped cutting herself (self-injury) and began loving herself at about age twenty, when she became Ginger and no longer had to submit to being called and classified as George. At this point in her life she feels that "I know who I am and people accept me for who I am." Shortly before writing this chapter, we were sitting with Ginger over a cup of coffee. She had recently been placed into temporary housing in a rooming house near Susan's home, a proximity that absolutely delights

Ginger (and Susan). Repeating (for the umpteenth time since we had met her) the stories of the boys who used to beat her up when she was growing up, and how she left home to protect her family and younger brother, Ginger added with a great deal of relish: "Now when I go back to the old neighborhood, the boys who used to beat me up are junkies, in jail, or dead."

On many levels Ginger has helped us understand that while drugs can be useful for some people sometimes, drugs—licit and illicit—can often both be a symptom of problems and make problems worse. The young thugs in her working-class neighborhood turned to heavy drug use at a time when economic restructuring caused many Americans to feel discouraged, to feel that they were losing out on the American Dream, but today they are "junkies, in jail, or dead." Ginger was given drugs by doctors and sought street drugs, in her assessment, to "self-medicate" the misery that she experienced because of sexism and homophobia. But drugs led her into prostitution, jail, and far too many assaults when she was too strung out to escape or fight back.

While much of Ginger's life has been lived in the sexist, racist, and homophobic purgatories of psychiatric hospitals, streets, and prisons, at this point in her life she has come to understand that her problems do not lie with her own pathology or bad choices but rather with social attitudes, practices, and policies that define her as sick or criminal. She is one of the only project women to have ever mentioned politics. Although her grasp of the details was a bit garbled, she was thrilled when Elizabeth Warren was elected to the Senate, "because Elizabeth will let gay people get married." Like several of the black women who participated in this project (Tonya in particular), Ginger senses that her suffering was caused by outside forces (namely, homophobia and anti-transgender discrimination, as well as the racism she is subjected to because her husband is black). Having attended events organized by a local transgender activist organization, she has come to learn that her own inadequacies as a man or as a woman are not the cause of her suffering. And she is sufficiently bighearted, if not to forgive the thugs, at least to understand that they beat her because that is what "society" (her word) expected them to do.

Like all of us, Ginger is a study in contradictions. She is equally comfortable these days unshaven and in jeans or made up and in a miniskirt and high heels. She has decided against taking female hormones because she has heard that they can cause breast cancer (her mother has cancer, so this is a deep concern for Ginger), she no longer spends her money on crack (she no longer feels the need to "self-medicate"), and she has stopped therapy and gone off psychiatric medication (she feels that she has seen therapists and psychiatrists "forever" and "enough is enough"). But she lets us know that she is not done with *all* medicalized solutions. A highlight of Ginger's year is the annual Boston Gay Pride Parade. Typically she begins planning what she'll wear to the parade a good two months in advance. This year she stopped by our office a month or so before the parade. Complaining that the hormones she had taken earlier had caused her to "get a belly" (to our eyes, just the slightest pooch—Ginger has remained slim her entire life), she showed us the diet pills she had just purchased at the pharmacy down the street from our office.

CHAPTER 5

"It's All in My Head"

Suffering, PTSD, and the Triumph of the Therapeutic

Many oppressed persons come to regard themselves as uniquely unable to satisfy
normal criteria of psychological health or moral adequacy
—Sandra Bartky, *Femininity and Domination* (1990)

"I'm doing better," Gloria told us; "I realized my issues are all up in my head."
Over a period of weeks preceding this realization she had complained about
the "dude" in her rooming house who was stalking her, knocking on her door
in the middle of the night, and lurking in the hallway outside her room. She
had pointed the man out to us. We had seen him staring at her and making
threatening and suggestive gestures, and we had heard him call out the window
to her with a demand for sex. Why, we wondered, was Gloria now saying that
her "issues" had to do with her own head rather than with the actions of the
"dude"?

An African American woman in her early fifties, Gloria grew up in a working-
class family in one of Boston's racially segregated neighborhoods. Her father
worked a blue-collar government job; her mother held a pink-collar job in
the private sector. The youngest by several years, Gloria is the only one among
the siblings in her family without a job, stable housing, and a stable
family. Gloria is not sure why that is so, but she thinks maybe "it's because of
the crack." Unlike her older siblings, Gloria came of age during the second
half of the 1980s when crack cocaine was introduced into America's
urban ghettos. Although Gloria does not point this out, these are the same
years in which economic recession, decline in the manufacturing sector,

and job flight from urban neighborhoods led to high unemployment and a generation of young African Americans who found it increasingly difficult to be hired.

Shortly after graduating high school, Gloria gave birth to her first son. "His father was not a good dad," she told us, and Gloria continued living with her mother, who helped take care of the baby. With few job opportunities available, Gloria took shifts "dancing" (stripping) at a bar down the street from her parents' apartment. "It had always been there, and everyone knew they paid good money—$75 a night." In the beginning, she recalls, it was "uncomfortable," but she liked to dance and as she got to know the customers, she felt more at ease. At about that time she met a man who gave her one hit of a crack pipe. From that first hit, Gloria reminisces, "I loved it. Then more and more." "Why did you start to use crack?" we asked. "I just plain liked being high on crack. I got into crack because I liked it too much." "Was this during the days in which crack was everywhere?" we asked. "Oh, yes! People were cooking it up in their apartments."

A year or so later Gloria fell in love with a man who tried to pimp her. She ran away when the man "put his hands on me." She recalls that when he beat her up in a park, she "yelled for help," but no one came to her assistance. Throughout her twenties and thirties her life revolved around crack—getting it and smoking it. When on drug runs (periods in which she used drugs intensively) she generally stayed with male friends, but her mother's apartment was always a safe place where she could go in order to rest and regain her strength. Her father died in 1990, and when her mother became sick in 2000, Gloria took care of her while she was ill and dying. When her mother died, Gloria was told to leave the government-subsidized apartment that was rented in her mother's name. For Gloria her mother's death was an important turning point. Before her mother died, "I always had a roof over my head."

Several years later Gloria suffered an assault that changed her life even more profoundly. In the wake of a drug deal gone wrong, she was jumped. During the attack she suffered a traumatic head injury that caused chronic memory loss. After two years in the hospital and a rehabilitation facility where she received treatment for brain injury and PTSD, she was released to the streets and was homeless, with the expectation that she would get by on her SSI payment of less than $700 a month.

No longer able to earn a living, for the next ten years Gloria moved in and out of homeless shelters, the apartments of male acquaintances (in return for sex), crack houses, and occasional overnights at her son's grandmother's apartment.

———————

A slim woman (sometimes too slim when she is on a crack run), Gloria delights in elaborate wigs, stylish hats, designer jeans (or knock-offs thereof), and faux leather and fur jackets. With a ready smile, despite the chaos in her living arrangements and her ongoing struggles with cognitive tasks, Gloria stayed in touch with us throughout the five years of the project. Often, we met her at Dunkin Donuts, where she'd sip a large tea, praise us for refraining from the doughnut shelf, and glance nervously out the window, hoping that none of the men who pressure her for sex would approach us.

During the time we have known Gloria, her greatest concern has been housing. Without a stable place to live, she is dependent on men, vulnerable to assaults on the streets, and visible to police who regularly stop her for loitering, soliciting, or simply "walking while black." Shortly after we first met her, she was placed in an SRO (single-resident occupancy) building by an agency that helps the homeless. Gloria was delighted finally to have a room of her own with her very own key, and she appreciated the caseworker who came by on a regular basis to make sure that she was taking responsibility for paying her bills. But within a year the downsides of this rooming-house arrangement became clear. She shared a bathroom, did not have access to a kitchen, and could not host overnight guests (not even her children). Most troubling, she learned that because she now had a room, "I am low on the [priority] list for a [government-subsidized] apartment because they are giving them first to homeless people and I have a place. . . . I am upset with myself. I should have worked with [another agency that places homeless people into apartments]." After asking around, we learned that clients are allowed to work with only one agency at a time—the SRO agency or the apartment agency. An apartment is more desirable than a room in an SRO, but the process for obtaining a subsidized apartment typically takes many years, while placement in an SRO tends to be a much shorter process. We have never heard Gloria question why homeless people like her are forced to choose between these two agencies (much less why some people are homeless when other people live in big houses with multiple empty bedrooms). She occasionally raises the possibility that she suffers because of "messed up" rules. Typically, however, she focuses on herself as the true source of her problems, saying that she "chose" to work with the wrong agency and that "even my caseworker says I need to work on myself first."

Like many other buildings of its kind, the SRO is populated both by disabled adults and by junkies and drug dealers. From the start Gloria was afraid of "the dude upstairs," who would stand outside her door, sometimes knocking, sometimes listening through the space around the threshold, sometimes sneaking up on her when she came out of the (shared) bathroom. Upset by his stalking, she told us, "I need to see a therapist." On occasion Gloria told us that she believed she was "hearing voices," while at other times she let us know that she was sure they were "real voices from outside my door." The "dude," who lived directly above her in her SRO, stalked her for close to two years. Typically, after describing how "the dude stands outside my door day and night," she would add, "But I think it's really my own paranoia. . . . I have crazy thoughts. I have this thing about men." While we are committed to presenting the Boston women's experiences in their own terms, we feel compelled to acknowledge that we have met this neighbor several times; he does exist, he does come over to Gloria and say inappropriate things, and the SRO building manager has seen these interactions but has not evicted the "dude." Although we were not able to know what happened outside our presence, we can note that on one occasion when we were chatting on the front steps of the SRO, a male tenant in the building called to tell her to come to his room, that he had crack, "and we'd better fuck."

If housing was Gloria's biggest worry, men were a close second. Several years after Gloria moved into the SRO, her boyfriend, John, was released from prison. Like many men exiting prison, he did not have any place to live and, because of his criminal record, was essentially unemployable. Although Gloria could have been evicted for hosting an overnight guest, John insisted on coming to stay with her. Gloria's concerns were grounded in her own history. A decade earlier she had been evicted from her apartment in public housing for "harboring a fugitive" (that is, a boyfriend who had an outstanding warrant for failure to meet with his parole officer was staying with her). Within days of moving in with her, John returned to using drugs and stealing things (including money from Gloria). Over the next few weeks Gloria told us that she was worried; "I get suspicious of him all the time. I know this is crazy but I can't stop the thoughts coming into my head. [For example] if he goes to the bathroom [the shared bathroom in the hall of the rooming house], I think he is having sex with the dude who lives upstairs." Still, "he is the best man I've ever been with. He makes me feel loved. He hugs me on the street."

A few months after moving in, John smacked her in the face, poured water on her head, and locked her in her room. A few weeks later he threw her against the wall. She called the police and went to the emergency room, where the medical staff gave her Ibuprofen and sent her home. She didn't file a complaint against John, because she didn't want to make him angrier. Not long afterward he smashed her cell phone so that she would not be able to call her friends or family, and he threatened that if she broke up with him, she would "have nothing." Nearly every time we spoke over the next year or so, Gloria voiced her fears of John and the "dude," as well as her fear that maybe the problem was her own "paranoia," not their behavior. While the broken cell phone, facial bruises, catcalls out the window, and John's many arrests suggest that John really is hurting her and the dude really is stalking her, Gloria remains ambivalent about the causes of her misery.

After two years of threats and violence John moved out. However, he seemed to have obtained a key to her room and would sneak in when Gloria was out and throw her clothes and other personal items out the window. One night when she heard him standing outside her window, she called the police, who made a cursory search of the backyard and then left. The next day she called her caseworker at the agency that had placed her in the SRO. She was told that the agency did not have another housing option available for her at that time. She was, however, urged to follow up with the therapist whom the caseworker had recommended as part of her rehabilitation program.

FROM SUFFERING TO PTSD

Despite the miseries with which they live, most of the women we have come to know profess the belief that "normal" people lead happy lives in nice homes with loving families. Like Gloria, nearly all the Boston women have been in and out of individual and group therapy for years or even decades. Many were sent as children to therapists as the first and sometimes sole response to abusive family situations. Virtually all of the women are conversant with terms such as *battered women's syndrome, PTSD, bipolar, codependence, low self-esteem, masochism,* and *"being in denial."* All have been in self-help therapeutic programs such as Alcoholics Anonymous (the theme of chapter 6). Requirements to attend AA and NA (Narcotics Anonymous) meetings and therapy sessions are common for women on probation or parole and for women who are involved with Child Welfare Services as a condition to see or keep their children. Many have been treated in in-patient hospital settings and have seen therapists while in prison.[1] And virtually all of the women spend large amounts of time, especially while in prison, watching television shows such as *Jerry Springer* and *Oprah* that implicitly and explicitly rehearse psychotherapeutically informed scripts that mock women for masochistically choosing to stay with cheating men (*Jerry*) or encourage women to develop the self-esteem to leave abusive men (*Oprah*).

The message they pick up from the many therapists who have treated them, the many therapeutic groups in which they have participated, and the pop therapeutic experts they see on television shows is surprisingly consistent: you suffer because of your personal unresolved traumatic experiences, emotional weaknesses, and character flaws, and the way to address your suffering is through therapy and medication.[2] In the context of our contemporary American grand narrative of individual responsibility, a person who experiences abuse, poverty, homelessness, incarceration, or even illness is likely to feel that there is something wrong with her, not with society.

The *Diagnostic and Statistical Manual of Mental Disorders* (DSM), published by the American Psychiatric Association, is the standard text used in the United States for defining and classifying mental disorders. First published in 1952 and then revised at approximately ten-year intervals, the *DSM* comprises categories used by doctors, therapists, insurance companies, and the correctional system. Each subsequent version of the *DSM* expanded the number of symptoms it included as indicating mental illness. It is critical to understand that psychiatric diagnoses are not objective descriptions of scientifically verifiable pathological markers in the way that medical diagnoses such as cancer or infection are.[3] There are no independent empirical tests for determining whether an individual has depression, anxiety disorder, PTSD, or any other psychological disorder, or even whether these are factually discreet categories. Despite this, the DSM definitions "have become the authoritative arbiter of what is and is not considered a mental disorder throughout our society" (Horwitz & Wakefield 2007, p. 7). Put bluntly, "psychiatric diagnosis can be understood as functioning as a political device, in the sense that it legitimates a particular social response to aberrant behavior of sorts, but protects that response from any democratic challenge" (Moncrieff 2010, p. 371).

In a recent essay, Marcia Angell (2011), former editor-in-chief of the *New England Journal of Medicine*, expressed concern regarding expanded pathologizing of normal behavior and overdiagnosis of psychiatric disorders. When normal sadness is treated as a depressive disorder, it becomes difficult to recognize the relationship of sadness to adverse social conditions and to identify appropriate social interventions. In fact, several decades of research indicate that some of the most consistent associations between social context and sadness do not stem from acute situations of loss but rather from chronic social stressors such as long-term unemployment, chronic physical illnesses, subordinate positions in family and interpersonal hierarchies, troubled marriages, and oppressive work situations. And studies show that when people move from chronic impoverished conditions to relatively more prosperous ones, their levels of distress fall (Horwitz and Wakefield 2007, p. 37).

Since the publication of the first edition of the *DSM*, according to Allan Horwitz and Jerome Wakefield, experiences that were, throughout history, understood as normal sorrow and sadness have become transformed into diagnosable disorders. With each diagnostic expansion of the *DSM*, more expressions of suffering and more sufferers become caught in the net of pathology. In 1980, for the first time, the *DSM* (in its third incarnation) included posttraumatic stress disorder (PTSD) as an official diagnostic category. Over the ensuing decades PTSD rapidly became the dominant framework for understanding and addressing suffering in America. Nearly all of the Boston women have been diagnosed with and treated for PTSD, and we heard PTSD invoked in many of the settings they frequented: homeless shelters, prisons, psychiatric hospitals, and even churches.

PTSD has proven to be something of a double-edged sword. Recognition of PTSD as a legitimate condition liberated former soldiers whose flashbacks and dysfunctions had earlier been seen as either cowardice or malingering, and it liberated raped and battered women from accusations of hysteria, hypochondria, actually having "enjoyed it," or having made false allegations in order to get back at men. However, while a PTSD diagnosis acknowledges that something bad really has happened to the individual, the response PTSD calls for is engagement with one's personal reaction rather than with the underlying issues of war or structural violence that created the conditions that gave rise to the suffering.

The focus on the particular individual's response to trauma draws attention away from the structural inequalities that give rise to a great deal of suffering.

In the case of sexual assaults such as those suffered by Gloria, Francesca, and others, this response "creates a fundamental assumption that a rape or sexual battery is an isolated traumatic event," rather than a consequence of structural inequalities (Bumiller 2008, pp. 91–92). In a similar vein, Fassin and Rechtman (2009) observe that impoverished black men and women in New Orleans after Hurricane Katrina were labeled and cared for as worthy victims of an unexpected trauma. Pre-Katrina, of course, many of those same people were poor, lived in substandard housing, had high rates of chronic and acute illnesses, and were more likely than white or affluent people to be stopped and frisked, arrested, or locked up. But that suffering was not legitimized by being called trauma by powerful psychiatrists.

Shortly after being assaulted, hospitalized for her injuries, and then released from the hospital back into homelessness, Elizabeth (chapter 2) shared with us that her therapists and caseworkers were telling her that she uses her past trauma as an excuse for not functioning well in the present time. But, Elizabeth said, she does not think trauma is "just" an excuse when she struggles daily with the ongoing dangers of homelessness and assaults on the street. While a PTSD diagnosis legitimizes women's claims that assaults and abuse really did take place (and are not a Freudian fantasy), it opens the door to medicalization—to bringing in doctors, radiologists, and psychiatrists to "prove" that women really have been hurt (Fassin & Rechtman 2009; see also Furedi 2004). In medicalized cultures like our own, doctors boast a scientific expertise and an aura of objectivity that few other professions can claim.[4] Physicians are employed to control and supervise those deemed to be deviant, to adjudicate punishment in carceral institutions, to justify insanity defenses, and to decide who is mad and who is bad—who is helped (treated) and who is punished. In perhaps the most extreme example of the synergy of medicalization and criminalization, physicians are called upon to administer lethal injections to death row inmates. With the authority to determine SSDI and SSI eligibility, physicians are gatekeepers for the range of services on which poor and disabled Americans depend in order to survive. The successive editions of the DSM have been used as the final authority in determining whether insurance will cover treatment and whether schools will provide support services. With the power to determine who is merely a drug seeker and who is a "legitimate" pain patient, the physician is "set up as an arbiter of the moral order" (Bell & Salmon 2009, p. 174). Equally if not more important, utilizing physician-documented illness as the justification for social benefits for certain people allows us as a society to avoid talking about basic human *rights* to minimum standards of food, housing, health care, and safety—a collective framework—and instead to talk about *need*—an individualistic framework implying weakness (cf. Stone 1979).

Although some visits with doctors and therapists are not voluntary but are rather required by a program or are necessary for obtaining disability benefits, the Boston women often eagerly sought medical and therapeutic appointments. For some of the women, the appeal of doctors and therapists lay in the one-on-one attention, a rare commodity on the circuit of homeless shelters and prisons. In a world in which not many people respect or even see the suffering of marginalized women, doctors and therapists may acknowledge that their suffering, at least on some level, is real. We heard from Elizabeth, Francesca, and others a sense of validation when the doctor recorded a diagnosis of PTSD or another official disease, especially when the doctor said that the problem was genetic or biological. Medical explanations seem to offer absolution. Going to the doctor feels like (and the women were told it is) "doing the right thing," or at least taking some sort of proactive step.

Mainstream psychotherapy treats PTSD as a normal reaction to trauma, and the therapeutic community does not condemn the individual for those reactions. Still, clients are taught that these adaptations to trauma are no longer necessary in the present, that prolonged PTSD is a failure to deal with trauma in a positive way, that the goal of therapy is to learn to adapt to the new circumstances and to recognize that fear, hypervigilance, and fight-or-flight hyperarousal are no longer necessary and may even be harmful to daily life. If the issue is psychological or emotional, one should be able to get over it with the right help.[5] In a culture that expects medicine to alleviate suffering, individuals who do not overcome afflictions may be scorned, stigmatized, or punished. However, for Gloria, as for many other women, threats to safety and well-being are current, real, and omnipresent. There is little sense in treating Gloria to "get rid of" PTSD adaptations, because they are *still* useful; being hypervigilant when you are homeless or being stalked can save your life.

Echoing the notion that the problem lies inside the individual and not with the outside world, the women of this project typically describe themselves as personally flawed rather than as victims of gendered, racial, and economic inequalities. A year or so into her saga of the SRO Gloria met us for coffee at a neighborhood Dunkin Donuts. When we commented that she seemed less distressed than she had been the previous time we talked, she explained that she felt calmer "because I realized my issues were all up in my head and I have stopped going there." The "issues" she referred to were, as we knew, the "dude" living upstairs who was stalking her in the real SRO, not in her head. On another occasion she told us, "Relationships, men, are the thing [problem] with me. I have crazy ideas about men. . . . I don't like to be by myself but I make bad choices in men." Similarly, in the context of talking about her boyfriend who went missing, Tonya, an African American woman, mused, "It's me in my head. . . . My man went missing for a couple of days and I was really worried. Afraid he was locked up. I started panicking over not having money. And when I panic I start having chaotic thinking." Knowing Tonya well, we knew that she really did not have any money, and we knew that her fear that her man was locked up was realistic considering the mass incarceration of black men in America. (Indeed, it turned out that he was in jail.)

In an odd sleight of hand, psychotherapeutic diagnoses both take away certain aspects of individual experience and individualize the collective suffering of racism, sexism, and poverty. If X happened to you, then you are now Y, and your decisions and personality traits boil down to PTSD, codependence, or (fill in the diagnosis here); the focus is now the diagnostic category rather than the unique individual or the social reality. A psychiatric diagnosis may destigmatize the individual's problems, but it also eliminates the possibility of seeing valor or meaning in suffering. Fassin and Rechtman (2009, p. 281) argue that "trauma obliterates experiences. It operates as a screen between the event and its context on the one hand, and the subject and the meaning he or she gives to the situation on the other hand."

GLORIA

A few years after we first met, Gloria's drug use spun out of control. She fell behind in her rent, she was spending far too much time with men who used her for sex in return for hits of crack, she lost a great deal of weight, and her conversations with us sounded confused. Her adult sons and sisters picked her up at her SRO, took her to stay with family for a few weeks, and then brought her to a drug rehab program for women. At many such rehab facilities, an organized daily routine of chores and meetings is designed to teach women about schedules and structure. Residents are not permitted to leave the premises even to see their children and are limited in their use of the telephone. They attend multiple therapy, group therapy, and Twelve Step meetings every day. The program demands a high level of personal account-ability regarding rules; encourages the women to "work on themselves" in terms of dealing with resentment, disappointment, frustration, anger, and sadness; and supports "spiritual growth."

A few days after leaving rehab, Gloria stopped by our office to share her excitement about the program. We asked her why this particular program had worked for her. After a bit of thought she shared this example: "In one group they asked about bad things that happened in our childhoods. I said I couldn't think of anything. The counselor told me that I am blocking some-thing. But I didn't remember any bad things. Then I heard a voice in the room say 'abandonment' and I thought, 'Yes, that is it!' God was showing me [through this voice] that is the thing I am blocking." Gloria had never before mentioned to us that she had been abandoned as a child; quite the contrary, she often described growing up as the beloved baby sister in a large close-knit family. On more than one occasion she had told us that her mother and father "were the best parents ever—they stuck it out 'til death do us part.'" So we asked her to explain the abandonment. "Yes. I didn't understand, either," she said. "So after I left the program, I called my older sister. She said I was the cutest baby and that they all had a rotation taking care of me, and that when they took me out in my stroller, everyone would come over and say how cute I am." With growing doubt regarding the "abandonment" idea, Gloria went on to call each of her older sisters in turn, and each told her the same thing: as the youngest of eight siblings she was coddled and never neglected or aban-doned. "My sister said it was my lifestyle that brought me to drugs, not my childhood."

REHABILITATING WOMEN'S PATHOLOGIES

The mantras that Gloria learned in the program were not new; she had been taught them numerous times before in women-centered or gender-sensitive programs for addicts, inmates, and other unfortunate women. E. Summerson Carr (2011), a linguist, analyzed the language used in a rather typical "gender sensitive" women's addiction treatment program. Both counselors and female clients talk about women's drug use in terms of early childhood victimization rather than adult poverty, homelessness, or race-based discrimination. Women are taught a therapeutic language that they need to adopt in order to be deemed recovered and gain access to housing and other critical resources. In Carr's observations, women clients often felt they had to connect their drug use to early sexual abuse in order "to meet their therapists' implicit demands . . . as few other plot lines were considered legitimate" (2011, p. 115).

While in rehab Gloria participated in a group on "how to lose the victim mentality." This was not the first time Gloria heard that script. *Oprah,* Twelve Step groups, therapists, judges, and correctional officers routinely advise women like Gloria to "stop being a victim," as if her victimhood is somehow a choice that she has made. These accusations echo wider cultural views in which being a victim—as opposed to being a survivor—tends to be seen as a sign of giving up, of failing to take responsibility for one's own self-preservation. The script of individual responsibility holds enormous power over institutional captives. Poor and criminalized women may be required to "own up" to their failings in the presence of judges (especially in drug courts), probation and parole officers, doctors, therapists, and caseworkers. Proper recitation of such confessions may be rewarded with custody of children, appropriate medical treatment (rather than the label "drug seeker"), reinstatement of welfare eligibility, a police warning (rather than an arrest), or probation (rather than incarceration).

Drawing on fieldwork in woman-centered programs in prison, Lynne Haney (2010, p. 117) argues that, "with its emergence in carceral settings, the therapeutic has clearly become a mode of state punishment. In addition to offering a template to make sense of the world, therapeutics serves as a technique of governance, used to manage psychological and emotional conduct in ways that align with the aims of government." In 1992, when Haney carried out her initial research, the dominant program ideology construed women's problems in terms of their need for education and job training so that they could be self-reliant and independent of government assistance. In line with neoliberal ideas of personal responsibility, women were encouraged to take responsibility for their choices and their lives (while absolving the state of responsibility for living wages, affordable housing, etc.). By 2002, Haney found, the emphasis had shifted to a purely psychotherapeutic model. Dismissing structural factors of any sort, counselors emphasized that all women in the program were addicts even if they didn't use drugs. Declared to be addicted to male attention, abuse, overeating, and so on, the women were instructed to take responsibility for the consequences of problems such as poverty and male violence—problems largely outside their control (on the ideological practices of women's drug treatment programs, see McCorkel 2013).

In therapeutic programs, women like Gloria are taught *both* that they need to take responsibility for their lives *and* that because of childhood traumas and feminine inclinations, they are fundamentally incapable of taking that responsibility. Perhaps the most disturbing message that emerges from program rhetoric and practices is that the line between women's illness and women's criminality can be confusingly vague. Throughout the institutional circuit, women are seen as especially likely to suffer from physical and emotional pathology, and female criminality is seen as gender deviance—whereas male criminality is more or less just exaggerated maleness. Women are given the message that there is something wrong with "you," singular, personally, whereas male criminality is more or less "normal." Women are told that, unlike men, they as women use drugs for psychological reasons of self-medication such as numbing their PTSD symptoms. In contrast, for men, drug use and criminality are often interpreted as a means of proving oneself to the gang or simply an expression of male nature.

We see the characterization of women's criminality in terms of women's pathology as part of a much larger cultural theme portraying women as damaged or, at least, especially vulnerable to damage. Women are prescribed antidepressant and anti-anxiety medication at far higher rates than men. And women's routine bodily functions are targeted for medical intervention. Prime examples include premenstrual syndrome (PMS) diagnoses, hormone replacement therapy (HRT), and cesarean sections performed at rates as high as 40 percent in parts of the country.

———

"Empowering women" was a catchphrase in many of the therapeutic settings frequented by the Boston women (at least during the five years of our project). While we inferred that "empowerment" is a good thing (certainly better than "disempowerment"), we are far from convinced that coerced therapy in prisons and rehabilitation centers can actually "empower" anyone. More broadly, "empowering" someone else in and of itself is an expression of a power relationship. If anything, the therapist has power over a model that defines health and illness, with health being defined as the ability to make choices and set goals to reach desired outcomes—actions that many people cannot accomplish because of external constraints (Dana Becker 2005). For women like Gloria, for whom therapy is part of a broader program of rehabilitation, the therapist typically works within a hierarchical organization; thus the power over the client is both the power of the particular therapist and the power of the broader organization.

Our argument is not that therapy is not a useful tool in the arsenal of approaches to dealing with human misery. Our concern is with the triumph of the therapeutic—with the (near) monopoly of psychiatric and psycho-therapeutic responses to suffering. Therapy has a place, but it can't solve structural problems. We suspect that therapy is more likely to be effective for securely housed middle-class Americans whose lives are more or less "working" except for particular emotional or psychological problems. For people strug-gling with poverty, insecure housing, violence, and social exclusion, therapy needs to be part of what Mary Harvey (2007, p. 16) calls "ecologically informed intervention at individual, community, and societal levels."

We wonder about the impact of the therapy in which the women have volun-tarily and involuntarily participated, in many cases for decades. In much of the country mental health care (along with oral health care) is treated as the unwanted stepchild of the health care system. Even in Massachusetts, where laws mandate parity between mental and physical health care in terms of insurance, the women of this project have seen hundreds of psychologists, counselors, social workers, and psychiatrists as they themselves have shuffled from facility to facility both in and out of jail, and as health providers in community mental health clinics and other facilities serving the poor and homeless have rapidly burned out and moved on to other jobs (the pay is low, and working with clients who need housing while all that the therapist can offer is talk is incredibly stressful). What often is described as a revolving door of clients can also be, from the client's perspective, a revolving door of therapists. Donna, a white woman in her forties, explains: "It's really a pain starting all over again with a new therapist. You tell the same story over and over again to different people. Then they leave and you start over again." More than one woman told us that she does not tell new therapists all of the horrible things that have happened, because, in Kahtia's words, "I don't want to upset her; I don't think she could handle it. My last therapist never called me back when I left messages with her trying to make a follow-up appointment." Since one of the strongest predictors of therapeutic success lies in the therapeu-tic alliance, therapist roulette is unproductive at best and damaging at worst when the therapeutic relationship of trust is repeatedly broken (cf. Harvey 2007). Opening deep wounds that the women have learned to deal with can be too high a price to pay when the therapy is abruptly and prematurely terminated.

Does repeatedly discussing how one is dealing with one's personal traumas keep alive the emotional impact of incidents that happened decades ago? Ethan Watters (2010, pp. 65ff.) believes talk therapy to have had such an effect when the American mental health personnel who descended en masse on Sri Lanka after the 2004 tsunami insisted that, in order to be healed, Sri Lankan adults and children needed to tell and retell the horrors they had experienced. Health workers pursued this therapy despite the established Sri Lankan belief that talking about horrors keeps them alive, despite Sri Lankans' clear preferences to get on with physical and social rebuilding rather than talking and analyzing, and despite their requests for food and building supplies rather than psychiatric medication. We Americans tend to take on faith that "talking things through" and "not holding things in" is healthy. The Boston women's experience, however, suggests that constantly discussing the past reinvigorates the emotional impact of incidents that happened decades ago, and that hearing about other women's problems in support groups further triggers a woman's own distress. As Joy told us, "Therapy doesn't work. I've had therapy since age seven. . . . It makes it worse, rehashing the same shit." Melanie, a white woman in her late thirties, had been trying to see a therapist for six months. After finally arranging an appointment, she decided not to go, explaining that she felt she was in a good place right then and didn't want to stir up old problems. "Counseling makes me worse," she said. "It brings up old shit that I'd rather not think about. I don't like how therapists dig into your mind." And Tonya suggests that constantly talking about your problems keeps you stuck thinking about them, rather than moving on and actually enacting real change.

FROM WEAKNESS TO STRENGTH

Over the five years of our project, we learned how highly the women valued generosity, caring, caregiving, and kindness. In our initial conversations we asked the question, "What do you think is your best trait?" Nearly all of the women replied, "I am good-hearted, like to help people, great mother" (Francesca); "I am open, kindhearted, giving" (Robin); "I keep in contact with my family; I don't abuse them; I give them money when I get my check" (Vanessa); "I'm easy to talk to, a good listener, great mother" (Joy); "I have a good heart; I help anyone who needs help" (Elizabeth). Time and again, we have seen women share their last dollar or last cigarette with friends, acquaintances, or even complete strangers who looked to be in worse straits than they were. We have seen them care for their children with devotion and tenderness, and we have seen women who lost custody of their children care for the children of friends and relatives (cf. Collins 2000, esp. pp. 262ff.).

Ginger, the transgender woman whom we introduced in chapter 4, has survived repeated assaults while growing up in a conservative Irish Catholic neighborhood followed by two decades of working the streets largely due to her superb interpersonal skills and commitments. On a daily basis she visits or talks on the phone to her mother, aunt, and various cousins. Ginger has spent many nights sitting with her mother in the hospital and many days running errands, accompanying her mother to medical appointments, and keeping her company when she was too ill to leave the house. Ginger is also close to her brother and refers to his children as "my babies" and their mother as "my baby mama." She even moved to another state for several months to look after his toddler when he and his wife needed to put in long hours building up a small business. Ginger's long-standing relationships extend to her family of "girls like me," friends she described as "my gay mother," "my gay daughter," and "my gay sister." For the past fifteen years the members of her "gay family" have helped one another with money, a place to stay, and emotional support as well as cosmetic treatments, medication, and clothing. Ginger's superlative social skills have carried over into her relationship with us. She gives us Christmas presents (one year she gave Susan a Snuggie), she calls us at least once a week just to say hi, and makes a point of calling on our birthdays. She remembers the names and ages of our children and always asks after them. She has called to wish Susan's husband a happy Father's Day, a phone call that she reported (with pride) at least a half-dozen times to other women at the drop-in center. Yet at regular intervals Ginger announces that from now on "I need to do me" and that "my problem is that I am always looking after other people and taking care of them."

We find it troubling that the therapeutic groups and programs for women in shelters, prisons, and rehabilitation facilities focus on women's "unhealthy" propensity for caring more about relationships than themselves (cf. Chesney-Lind & Eliason 2006; Becker 2005; Pollack 2005). To "recover," the thinking goes, they must learn about their dysfunctions, addictions, dependencies and about battered women's syndrome and a host of other personal pathologies. Rehearsing these gendered scripts, the Boston women "confess" that their problems are caused by the fact that that they are "too nice" or "too generous" or "too focused on others and not on myself." Carly—a young, white woman, sexually abused as child, placed into the Child Welfare Services system, and homeless since leaving Child Welfare Services supervision at age eighteen— tells us, "My problem is I'm codependent and obsessed with sex." Kahtia's life has been filled with suffering since childhood, when her parents rented her out as a sex toy, followed by decades on the streets and loss of her children to Child Welfare Services (we share her experiences more fully in chapter 8). Kahtia on occasion attributed her suffering to what she saw as a typically feminine flaw: "My worst trait is that I am a caretaker; I'm a people pleaser." In Megan's words, "My problem is that I worry about how others are feeling, and I don't deal with my own issues." Elizabeth explains, "I am trying to get my life in order. I never concentrated on myself—it was always on my boy-friends."

The very thing that the women with whom we have been working believe they are good at and care deeply about—relationships—is interpreted as a symptom of pathology in institutional settings. We question the therapeutic efficacy of persuading women that their greatest strength is in fact not only a weakness but actually the cause of their victimization and suffering. The mes-sage that "your problem is that you are too generous" both negates the aspect of their being that most of the women see as most morally valuable and dis-courages women from building the webs of favors—borrowed and returned— that help them survive on the streets. And that, we believe, is therapeutically suspect.

CHAPTER 6

Higher Powers

*The Unholy Alliance of Religion, Self-Help
Ideology, and the State*

God grant us the serenity to accept the things we cannot change, courage to change
the things we can, and wisdom to know the difference.

—The Serenity Prayer (Alcoholics Anonymous World Services, Inc.)

When we first met Joy, she was so much the model resident of the halfway
house for women on parole that we informally pegged her as "most likely to
succeed" in the program. Enthusiastic about the counselors, the groups, the
classes, and the structure, she shared her optimism that she would stay drug
free and return to the middle-class lifestyle of her parents. The staff at the
facility was delighted with her "progress," and she was granted a great deal of
freedom to leave the building and see her father and daughter. Joy fluently
parroted the staff's Twelve Step language, talking of "recovery," "one day at a
time," "doing the right thing," and "turning myself over to God." Indeed, her
devotion to the program made it difficult for us to get a sense of who she was
aside from the iconic Twelve Step "addict."

Drugs have been both a source of consolation and of misery for Joy since she
was twelve years old. "Until I was seven, everything was normal—white picket
fence, father went to work, mother stayed home with the children. Then
everything fell apart." Her parents divorced, her mother received custody of
the children, and her mother's boyfriend molested Joy and her older sister for
the next five years. Her sister survived by throwing herself into figure skating
(though she did struggle with bulimia for several years) and moved away from

home as soon as she turned eighteen. Joy was treated by psychotherapists and prescribed psychiatric medication throughout her childhood. Her sister and her parents went to family counseling on and off as well.

Joy was removed from the home when Child Welfare Services put a 51A (an order to stay away) on her mother's boyfriend. Her mother chose to stay with the boyfriend, which meant that Joy had to leave. She went to live with her father (of whom she says, "He is wonderful, my best friend"), but in another stroke of misfortune, he had a heart attack a few days later. Although he survived, he was not sufficiently healthy to raise a troubled young girl on his own. At that point Joy went into the child welfare system and lived in various foster homes and juvenile programs. "None of these placements worked. I was an early drug abuser." Because of her behavioral issues she attended an alternative school for children with special needs. Still, "I was a fat freak. I never fit in." In bad shape from the molestation and abuse, and often a bit "zoned out" from psychiatric medicine, she had poor social skills, and other kids picked on her. She found the academics easy, but dropped out in the eleventh grade and turned her attention to crack cocaine.

During the ensuing twenty years there was no particular town that Joy considered home, though she has tended to move around among a handful of communities within a ten-or-so-mile radius of her father's house. During some periods, she has had a room in an SRO or halfway house. At other times she has been in jail, and in still other periods she has slept outside, even during New England winters. "I've been raped and beaten up and sodomized many times. . . . As a prostitute, I figured I asked for it—drugs had a hold on me." The worst attack occurred a year before we first met her. The perpetrator stabbed her in the uterus, she lost three and a half pints of blood, and she probably would have died if the police had not found her bleeding and unconscious on the street. "The police saved my life"—a sentiment that, Joy acknowledges, has much to do with her race (white) and her physical appearance ("cute").

Joy estimates that she has gone to the emergency room "maybe a hundred times in the last ten years, for things related to being homeless, being a prostitute." Now in her thirties she has a laundry list of past and current physical and emotional health challenges: asthma, digestive troubles, anxiety, diabetes, GERD (gastroesophageal reflux disease), hepatitis C, pelvic inflammatory disease, migraines, arthritis in the shoulder and hip (the legacy of various assaults), PTSD, bipolar disorder, depression, insomnia, cancer, and excruciating toothaches. She has been prescribed medication for all of these problems. Throughout her life she has been placed on myriad psychiatric medications. (Just during the time we have known her, she has been on Trileptal [seizure medication], Seroquel [depression, schizophrenia, and bipolar disorder], Abilify [depression, schizophrenia, and bipolar disorder], Remeron [depression], Buspar [anxiety], Celexa [depression], Wellbutrin [depression], Neurontin [seizures], and Effexor [depression and anxiety/panic disorder].) She has also completed dozens of detoxifications at dozens of different facilities, numerous inpatient stints, and the whole gamut of rehab programs. With a hint of bragging in her tone, she jokes that "I've been at [the local] hospital so many times they have a plaque for me!"

JOY ON THE TWELVE STEP CIRCUIT

A few months after we first met her, Joy disappeared from our radar. Week after week we asked friends, counselors, caseworkers, and family members to let her know if they saw her that we still cared about her and that she could stay in the project and receive the monthly incentive of a public transit pass, no questions asked. And then, out of the blue, she called to ask for a ride to court—a man who had raped her over a year ago was finally going to be tried. Looking very put-together in a new pair of shorts, a cute T-shirt, and recently cut hair, Joy was happy to see us. Since our last meeting, she explained, "I relapsed. Then I cleaned up. Then I relapsed again. Now I'm clean." After leaving the first rehab facility, she had moved in with a friend for a few weeks. "Then, things were very bad—I was on the streets in bad shape." She checked herself into a hospital with a unit for people with dual diagnoses (mental illness and drug addiction). The staff held her there for three weeks while stabilizing her medication and then arranged for her to move into a twenty-eight-day rehab program for women. When that ended, she had nowhere to go. She stayed with a friend for a while and then went back to the streets and to crack. Shortly before calling us, she had undergone another detox and moved into a "sober house," which is where we met up to drive to court.

Sober houses are meant to serve recovering addicts who are not quite ready to live on their own and could benefit from the structure and support of living with other former addicts. Many sober houses are loosely associated with AA or NA communities; AA/NA meetings may be held in the sober house, or sober house residents may go in groups to Twelve Step meetings. As a practical matter, men and women with criminal records often have trouble finding a landlord who will rent to them. A sober house, for women like Joy, is often the only alternative to the street or a strict and prohibitively expensive rehab facility. At some sober houses the residents are required to do urine tests; at others there is no such requirement. At some there are part-time caseworkers; others offer no special services. While there was no support staff at Joy's sober house, there was a good sense of camaraderie among the residents. Unfortunately, that camaraderie included sharing drugs.

When we arrived at the sober house to pick Joy up, we noticed a strange odor. This sober house, it turns out, was more of a crack house than anything else. Located on a side street across the way from a bar, the sober house looked like a two-family dwelling that had been turned into a boardinghouse. Several residents were sitting on the front stoop, smoking, drinking beer, and shooting the breeze. Inside, a warren of dark corridors was flanked by unmarked doors of residential rooms. An odor that we could not identify wafted through the corridors; that odor, Joy taught us, is the smell of a crack pipe. For the privilege of renting a single room with a shared bathroom and kitchen, Joy paid $680 per month. She would have liked to find a job, but between the bad economy and the sober house's isolated location, she had had no luck. She wanted to go back to the facility where we'd first met her, but was told that now they took only women on parole, and she had "wrapped" her period of correctional supervision. Joy asked us to help her put together an appropriate outfit for her court appearance. In an A-line skirt, printed button-down blouse, and subtle makeup, Joy drove with us to the courthouse and we sat down to wait. After several nervous hours she was told that the rape case had been continued to a future date. "Susan, I just want to stay clean. . . . I just can't live like this anymore. I'm worn out," Joy sobbed.

By summer, Joy's situation had deteriorated. When we stopped by the sober house to visit her for her birthday, we had to bang on the door of her room for a good five minutes to wake her up. She had been up crying hysterically for five hours the night before. People in the house had taken turns sitting with her, and they had even considered calling an ambulance. With a great deal of cajoling, she dressed and came out with us to get an ice cream cake (her favorite) to share with the other sober house residents. For the first time in our acquaintance Joy was not able to pull her appearance together. Stringy hair, haggard eyes, dingy clothing—this Joy bore little resemblance to the Twelve Step acolyte we had met earlier that year.

Away from the house Joy shared some of what had been going on. Her sister and nephews had come in from out of town to visit, but Joy's father would not let her see them until she gave him "clean" (drug-free) urine. However, at the time, she had been in a bad place emotionally and she used crack to, in her words, "self-medicate." By long-standing agreement with her father that she would stay away from her daughter when actively on drugs, she had not seen her family. On top of this, a month or so earlier her purse containing her ID had been stolen. After a long job search she was offered a job at a store near the sober house, but she needed her ID to take the job. She also couldn't get food stamps without her ID. She needed $15 to pay for a new ID, and her only income was SSI (see chapter 2), which was exactly enough to cover her rent, phone, and cable television (which she considered an absolute lifeline when she was too anxious to sleep at night).

A month later she was evicted from the sober house for getting into a loud argument with one of the "other girls" living in the house. Despite having left all her belongings behind—she had nowhere to store them—she was optimistic that this might be a "blessing in disguise," giving her the push to go to detox. "I'm doing the right thing. I'm happy," she told us when she phoned from the rehab facility that the detox staff had set up for her. (She initially was not allowed visitors.) "Susan, I am doing the right thing. For once I am happy. God puts me where He wants me to be." We talked about why she decided to stop using drugs, and she reminded us what terrible shape she had been in on her birthday. She felt as though she had "come to the end of the line" and "just couldn't do it anymore." More depressed than she had ever been in her life, "I had an epiphany and decided to go to detox." "How do you put your belief in God together with all of the horrible things that happen to you?" we asked her. "Sometimes I feel I deserve what happens for not taking care of my daughter." (Joy's daughter is happy, healthy, and well cared for by Joy's father.)

When we met in October, Joy was in an upbeat mood and was still delighted with the rehab facility. It was indeed lovely. A converted mansion surrounded by beautiful gardens, the house looked and felt like a country inn. Joy hoped to stay there for a year. She was proud of the house and showed us how she had decorated her room and bought pretty linens for her bed. Joy, like many of the other twenty "girls" (ranging in age from twenty-five to sixty, they are called girls) living in the house, had arranged stuffed animals on the bed and pictures of her daughter on the nightstand. Aside from the visual presence of her daughter, Joy's room could easily have been mistaken for a college dorm room, and Joy—in a cute ponytail—could have been taken for a slightly older than usual co-ed. At the rehab facility the women took turns cooking and learning life skills. The daily routine centered on Twelve Step meetings. "It's very helpful," Joy told us. "I learn to identify with other addicts instead of comparing myself to them and saying that I'm in better shape." Committed to staying off street drugs, Joy was faithfully taking her prescribed Trileptal (seizure medication), Buspar (anti-anxiety medication), and Celexa (an antidepressant). During her first few months in rehab she gained a significant amount of weight (she had lost a great deal of weight on her last drug run).[1] "I need OA [Overeaters Anonymous] or Weight Watchers. I stuff my feelings with food." Whenever we saw her during this period, she was on the upside of her mood swings. Ecstatic about the program and her sobriety, she had the intensity of a convert. We had to remind ourselves that in fact she had been through this process many times before; her current enthusiasm for recovery was nothing new.

––––––––––

Six months into the program it was time for Joy to start organizing her life beyond rehab. "I like it here. Everything is awesome. The staff is good. It's a good house. It lets you spread your wings, show you how to grow." With encouragement from the staff she enrolled in a training program to be a medical assistant. One month into the training she was calm, focused, and thrilled with her 4.0 GPA. We offered to take Joy out to the local Taco Bell to celebrate, and Francesca, who hadn't eaten for almost two days, asked if she could come along too. The contrast between the two women that day was dramatic. Francesca looked a wreck, carrying around her possessions in a ragged backpack, wearing a tank top that ended well above her navel, and sporting a new, infected tattoo on her neck. Joy had just gotten a nice haircut, with purple highlights done by a friend, and was wearing a pretty purple camisole under her shirt and a lovely pink lip gloss. A few weeks later she graduated from rehab and moved out.

Within a few months things started going downhill. It turned out that Joy had seven cavities, but she couldn't get them filled because she had maxed out her dental insurance coverage for the year. She could see her teeth rotting. "I used to say bad things about people with no teeth, and now I'm going to be one of them." She was struggling with the medical terminology class and began spending most of her time at AA/NA meetings. "I need to work on my recovery," Joy explained. "That needs to come first. Without recovery I can't move forward." A few weeks later Joy was so dedicated to "working on my recovery" that she was spending entire days at Twelve Step meetings rather than going to class. She dropped out four months shy of earning her certificate, owing $10,000 in student loans.[2] Then, at about ten months sober, "I relapsed. . . . There was a lot of shit going on, and I stopped going to meetings and networking and talking to people." By September she was no longer allowed to see her daughter. Her parents told us, "Joy is running hard on the streets."

Less than a year later Joy called to tell us that she was in detox again. "I realized that my only choices were to go hang myself or to try it again." This time, rehab was in a hospital setting where the detox ward was covered in notices announcing Twelve Step meetings and support groups. When we came to visit, Joy was sound asleep; the nurse didn't want to wake her, since she'd been up all night coming off crack. A week later Joy was gone. The detox staff could not find her a bed in rehab, so they discharged her onto the streets. Within a short time she wrecked the car of the friend with whom she had been staying and was arrested for trespassing when she went into the basement of a deserted house to change her clothes. She spent the next year in jail, on the streets, and occasionally staying with some trick for a few days or weeks. When we got together with Joy and Francesca for a cup of coffee, their roles had flipped since the previous gathering. Francesca was—for the time being—living fairly securely with her boyfriend Joey and her son. She was taking care of her health problems and planning a birthday party for her granddaughter, and Joey was in therapy and working on anger management. While Francesca shared recipes for some of the Italian classics she had cooked that week, Joy regaled us with stories of abuse at the hands of Tommy, her current boyfriend. "He's a dickhead. But people who live like me only attract dickheads." Joy put her fingers in an L-shape on her forehead, indicating that she was a "loser." Pulling an old idiom out of the recesses of her memory, she added, "If not for bad luck, I'd have no luck at all."

One warm June day, quite out of the blue, Joy called us. She was in a rehab program that didn't let her go off-site for doctors' appointments for the first six weeks, so she had not yet resumed her bipolar medication. She had not yet seen a therapist and had been crying a lot. Still, she was optimistic that in the long run this program would work for her. Unlike most programs that kick residents out for using drugs or drinking, this was a harm reduction program that allowed residents after the first six weeks to go to detox (if necessary) and come back. While much of the time in the program was unstructured, Twelve Step meetings were available nearly round the clock. Later, when Joy's six-week confinement was up, she met us at the women's center. Back in her bouncy ponytail, she earnestly preached to the other women (most of whom tuned her out): "I have a choice and I need to make the right choice. . . . I'm learning that I have a disease and I need God to help me be sober."

When she graduated from the rehab program, a bed was arranged for her at another facility, but both her Medicaid and Medicare had been cut off because mail sent to her at one of her former residences was returned "addressee unknown." Shortly afterward she managed to get her insurance back, but by that time there were no beds available. Joy went back to the streets, staying with male "friends" in return for sex. For the first time since we had met her, Joy was burned out on AA. "I don't have the desire to go. I can go to meetings, but then I have to go to the street to figure out where to live and that cancels out the hope."

Joy's anxiety about not having a place to go was well founded. A few weeks later she was attacked, beaten, and raped by a gang of men at a train station. Her ankle was fractured and her face was seriously bruised. The police finally came and took her to the hospital, where a rape kit was done. Joy decided not to press charges. "It's pointless with my history." In physical and emotional pain, she spent the next few weeks high.

Later that year we met Joy at a Dunkin Donuts near the apartment of a man with whom she had been staying. In our world Dunkin is a place you can go to sit with a friend over a cup of coffee. In this neighborhood there are no chairs or tables at Dunkin—"that's because they don't want the homeless people coming in," Joy explained. Looking cute in shorts, a T-shirt, and a ponytail, she was a bit stoned but very lively and focused. As we perched ourselves between the metal spikes on the low brick wall surrounding the Dunkin parking lot, Joy burst out, "I had a customer who turned out to be a policeman. He likes me and wants to expand the relationship, but I'm not interested. Remember Tommy? You met him before. Well, we've been together for a year. I really love him. I finally found a man who loves me back." With a job and an apartment, Tommy seemed much more stable than most of the men Joy had been involved with. Things were so good with Tommy that by Thanksgiving even her father recognized that this was a good relationship and invited Joy and Tommy to join the family for the Thanksgiving feast. Then, three days later, when Joy wouldn't go out and buy dope for him, Tommy beat her up, leaving her with a broken jaw. At the hospital her jaw was wired; she was given a day's worth of pain medication and then released.

A few months later Joy was back in detox, then in rehab in a holding program where she was waiting for a long-term placement somewhere else. "They just write something down [prescriptions] to shut you up. Don't take the time to listen to you. It's all about the money. We're a turnover. They kick you out when your insurance runs out." "How about the AA meetings," we asked her. "I'm grouped out. I could teach those classes."

ONCE AN ADDICT, ALWAYS AN ADDICT

THE TWELVE STEPS OF ALCOHOLICS ANONYMOUS

1. We admitted we were powerless over alcohol—that our lives had become unmanageable.
2. Came to believe that a Power greater than ourselves could restore us to sanity.
3. Made a decision to turn our will and our lives over to the care of God *as we understood Him.*
4. Made a searching and fearless moral inventory of ourselves.
5. Admitted to God, to ourselves, and to another human being the exact nature of our wrongs.
6. Were entirely ready to have God remove all these defects of character.
7. Humbly asked Him to remove our shortcomings.
8. Made a list of all persons we had harmed, and became willing to make amends to them all.
9. Made direct amends to such people wherever possible, except when to do so would injure them or others.
10. Continued to take personal inventory and when we were wrong promptly admitted it.
11. Sought through prayer and meditation to improve our conscious contact with God, *as we understood Him,* praying only for knowledge of His will for us and the power to carry that out.
12. Having had a spiritual awakening as the result of these Steps, we tried to carry this message to alcoholics, and to practice these principles in all our affairs. (A. A. World Services, Inc. Italics in the original.)

Virtually every Boston area drug treatment program includes a Twelve Step component. Both of the facilities where we initially met the Boston women host daily Twelve Step meetings and post Twelve Step information on bulletin boards and walls. The walls of many of the homeless shelters, halfway houses, soup kitchens, churches, clinics, sober houses, and rehab program rooms are plastered with AA slogans: "Don't feel sorry for yourself"; "Take responsibility"; "Everything happens as it should"; "Let go and let God"; "I can't . . . He can . . . I think I'll let Him (Steps 1, 2, 3)."

Alcoholics Anonymous and Narcotics Anonymous hold a uniquely institutionalized status within the institutional circuit and serve as the ideological core across institutions. Judges mandate AA/NA attendance for individuals accused or convicted of drunk driving or illegal drug use; drug courts routinely include AA/NA meetings as part of the program; AA/NA groups are held inside prisons and other correctional facilities; judges often require AA/NA attendance as a condition for contact with children or for parole (Sered and Norton-Hawk 2011b). While AA/NA participation is not obligatory in Massachusetts prisons, Twelve Step meetings are often the only regular opportunity to get out of the cells and socialize. Even more important, obtaining a certificate attesting to one's attendance at meetings can help one earn early release and prove to caseworkers that one is "doing the right thing." Throughout the circuit, women who need assistance with housing, food, health care, safety, or child care, as well as women drawn into the net of the correctional system, cannot avoid contact with and participation in Twelve Step programs. Although no systematic research documents how AA/NA became a mainstay of the institutional circuit, we suspect that the appeal of AA/NA lies in the Twelve Step resonance with the greater American metanarrative of personal responsibility, its Christian valence, and—perhaps more than anything else— its price: free. Run by volunteers, Twelve Step meetings are a fiscally conservative solution to suffering.

Founded in 1935 by "Bill W." and "Dr. Bob," Alcoholics Anonymous was an outgrowth of the Oxford Group, a Christian fellowship established some ten years earlier by the Lutheran minister Dr. Franklin Nathaniel Daniel Buchman. In contrast to the contemporaneous Progressive Era's Social Gospel movement's focus on economic inequality, the Oxford Group espoused the politically and theologically conservative view that suffering is caused by individual sinfulness. The Oxford Group's solution to sin and suffering lies in confession, taking individual responsibility for one's actions, and completely surrendering one's ego to God—conceived of as a powerful deity intimately involved in the affairs of this world (Mercadante 1996). With some softening of the overtly Christian language, AA applied these beliefs to recovery from alcoholism. On one level, AA/NA resonates with other medicalized responses to suffering: Twelve Step programs consistently refer to addiction as a "disease." At the same time, AA/NA echoes criminalized and religious responses to suffering: Twelve Step programs insist that addicts can choose to be abstinent through a process of turning themselves over to a Higher Power and engaging in an ongoing process of examining and owning up to one's "defects of character." Through slogans, readings, and personal testimony, AA/NA promotes the idea that one is responsible for one's failings, that happiness and healing can come only through admitting one's flaws and turning oneself over to a Higher Power, that blaming others for one's suffering is actually a symptom of the disease of addiction, and that it is either hubris or pathology to try to change the world.

Preaching that an addict is always an addict, a cure is not possible, and abstinence can be achieved only through following the Twelve Step program, AA/NA is a lifelong affiliation that demands loyalty on behalf of its members. Participation in AA/NA revolves around frequent meetings that combine recitation of the Twelve Steps and other credos with personal testimony regarding how one's life has been ruined by drink or drugs and how AA/NA helps one stay sober "one day at a time." In addition to meetings, AA/NA members are encouraged to speak daily with a lay sponsor (a more advanced recovering alcoholic or addict) and to systematically work through the Twelve Steps. For active participants, AA/NA provides an entire way of life and a social network. Members are encouraged to be loyal to the group and not critique the form or content (though they are encouraged to be critical of themselves). "Oh yes, in the beginning I resisted and my big ego got in the way," one participant has said, "but now I see they were right and I was wrong" (Kasl 1992, p. 39). The AA motto "Work it till it works" echoes American faith in the notion that hard work leads to (economic) success. Failure ("relapse") typically is construed as the failure of the *individual* to follow the program's rules faithfully. Long-term abstinence, in contrast, is considered proof of the *program's* success.

AA's iconic redemption stories in *The Big Book of Alcoholics Anonymous* (originally published in 1939) describe, for the most part, white middle-class men who had jobs, secure housing, and families—in other words, men for whom alcohol overuse threatened an otherwise happy, or at least socially normative, lifestyle. In AA's first decades, women were enlisted as a sort of ladies auxiliary for wives of alcoholic men (Tallen 1990). Today women participate as equal members in AA and predominate in some of the Twelve Step offshoots such as Overeaters Anonymous and Codependents Anonymous. According to one observer, Overeaters Anonymous's "program for self-stylization serves to reinscribe traditional gender values and configurations onto the eating-disordered woman, as she is slowly convinced that her resistance to the gendering (represented as false belief in personal power) is indeed what caused her eating disorder in the first place" (Lester 1999, p. 156). Bette Tallen (1990) has argued that the message of the codependency movement is that women should focus on themselves and not hold men responsible for violent and abusive behaviors. Codependents Anonymous helps people "live with the [social] system's failures. The group is not fostering individualism as much as it is helping people adjust when its promises fail them" (Irvine 1999, p. 160).[3]

There is little evidence beyond individual testimonies for AA's or NA's long-term success. Studies that claim effectiveness for AA/NA typically show a weak correlation between AA/NA attendance (especially frequent attendance) and abstinence during a relatively short period of time, but they fail to address causality—the fact that people who are actively using drugs or alcohol are less likely to attend AA/NA (Gossop, Stewart, & Marsden 2008; Kaskutas 2009; Nedderman, Underwood & Hardy 2010).[4] Given the omnipresence of Twelve Step programs and ideology in the correctional and substance abuse treatment world, and given the low rates of long-term abstinence among drug addicts, it is likely that current AA/NA attendees differ from nonattendees only in regard to the point in the "recovery-relapse" cycle that they happen to be in at the time of the study.

While Joy and a few others have had periods in which they were devout AA/NA members, none of the women we know sustained a commitment to the program for more than a couple of years. The AA/NA insistence that powerlessness is a personal feeling rather than a political reality, together with the Twelve Step emphasis on conformity, humility, and personal failings, is a poor fit for people who live with abuse, sexism, poverty, and other forms of oppression (Kasl 1992; Kaminer 1992; Tallen 1990). In response to our question, "What is the worst thing that has happened to you during the past few months?" the Boston women stress not having a place to live, arrest warrants hanging over their heads, physical and sexual assaults, not being allowed to see their children, and being estranged from their families. Many are bothered by AA/NA's insistence that their real problems are their attitudes, thoughts, and feelings rather than their lack of housing or the struggle to raise their children. Thus, at some point during almost all of our conversations with Elizabeth, she blamed herself for her lousy situation—that is, she faulted her procrastination, her bad choices, her inability to follow through with things she needs to do, her spotty attendance at AA meetings, and her laxity in calling her sponsor and reading the *Big Book*. Yet, in the very same conversations, she explained that "listening to other people's issues [at AA meetings] is not helpful. . . . To stop drinking I need a stable place to live so I won't worry all the time. . . . Drink calms down my racing thoughts." As for Gloria, her most pressing concerns for much of the time we have known her have centered on a violent and controlling boyfriend who orders her around, checks through her possessions to see what she is "hiding," and has even locked her in a room. "I don't want a sponsor," she explains. "I don't want someone telling me what to do."

It seems particularly egregious for women like Joy, Gloria, and Elizabeth to be reminded of their powerlessness when they confront the consequences of their lack of power on a daily basis at the hands of welfare and child service agencies, the courts, and violent men.[5] All of these women have already spent too much of their lives in the hands of too many higher powers; no matter how much they work on their own perceptions and reactions (which, according to Twelve Step ideology, are all that one can control), they remain vulnerable to powerful institutions and people. With its valorization of individual responsibility, Twelve Step ideology effectively places the blame on women whose poor health is a consequence of poverty, homelessness, and abuse and who have seen the men who rape them walk free because a judge or jury believed that a drug-using woman must be culpable in some way. When judges, doctors, and clergy all agree that addiction is a "spiritual disease" and that turning oneself over to a Higher Power is the solution, it is hard to avoid the message that if a woman does not "recover," the problem must lie with her own character defects (being "constitutionally incapable of being honest with themselves," as *The Big Book* says) and bad choices.

CHURCH AND STATE

Twelve Step meetings are characterized by standard religious attributes, including reference to the transcendent ("Higher Power"), encouragement of uncritical faith, sacred writings (the *Big Book*), rituals (recitation of the Twelve Steps and the Serenity Prayer), moral teachings, and a claim to unique truth. Rituals in general—such as confession, prayer, and sacrifice—imbue and reinforce beliefs, encouraging us to internalize, embody, and enact those beliefs so that they become experienced as part of the fiber of our being. As is most apparent in the ritualized greeting "I am So-and-so and I'm an alcoholic/addict," Twelve Step groups encourage members to take up an identity (recovering alcoholic/addict) congruent with that of the group (on interpellation and addict identity formation, cf. Aston 2009). The self-scrutiny and the public confession of pathology expected in Twelve Step groups are designed to lead the one who confesses into declaring a "truth" that she then is obligated to claim as her own.

Though not affiliated with any particular Christian denomination (and self-avowedly "spiritual," but "not religious), AA/NA echoes Christian theology and sensibilities: turning oneself over to God, confession, and the call to spread the word. About half of all Twelve Step groups meet in churches (often because they are the only community institutions that provide a free room for the meetings; generally the churches do not sponsor the meetings), and Christian ministers and pastors often recommend AA to congregants (Mercadante 1996). AA/NA encourages church attendance and has been shown to strengthen members' adherence to religious practice (Cahn 2005). While AA/NA officially insists that each member may have his or her own notion of a Higher Power, according to Isabella (whom we meet in chapter 8): "Every single person I've met [at meetings] means God by 'Higher Power.' They sometimes phrase it as 'My Higher Power, who I choose to call God,' but no one has any other kind of higher power." Indeed, nearly all of the women of our project invoke God ("turning it [my problem] over to God" and "thanking God for my sobriety") as an integral part of the Twelve Step program.[6]

The conservative Protestant emphasis on individual salvation articulated in AA/NA meetings is repeated on the institutional circuit, where many of the services, programs, and agencies that manage and treat criminalized and poor women are faith-based. Bibles and devotional tracts—together with inspirational Twelve Step mottos—are scattered throughout the halfway house where we initially met about half of the women. These women had been selected for early release from prison and were serving out their sentences on parole under the auspices of a Christian institution. Combining the language of Twelve Steps with that of Christianity, the halfway house's web page explains, "People in crisis often find comfort and stability in a higher power. Our spiritual offerings guide our program members through many ways to find healing through God." The facility offers prayer services, Bible study groups, AA and NA meetings, and counseling from a spiritual advisor. Attendance at prayer meetings is not mandatory, but residence at the facility requires compliance with rules formulated to shape the spiritual character of the residents. Women are regulated as to how often and how long one may shower, what to put on one's bed, when and where one has contact with men, what medication to take, and more important, what medication not to take (the mission does not allow "benzos"—the prescription anti-anxiety medication that most of the women feel they need to keep from being overwhelmed by fear and panic). In part because of the rigid regulation of day-to-day (and even minute-to-minute) behavior, many women do not finish the terms they were assigned in the halfway house as a condition for early release from prison, and instead "relapse" (in the language of AA/NA) and return to prison, where they may end up serving a longer stretch than had they simply finished out the prison term to begin with.

––––––

Overlaps among religion, medicalization, and criminalization are highlighted in the rapidly growing phenomenon of drug courts for handling individuals charged with low-level drug-related crimes. Currently more than 2,600 drug courts in the United States collectively handle the cases of more than 120,000 individuals each year (National Institute of Justice 2011; Brook 2010, p. 175), and the number of such courts and the number of people brought before them are growing as prisons have become too crowded and too expensive, and the public will to incarcerate drug addicts seems to be ebbing. Drug courts have been described as "resembl[ing] something between a revivalist meeting and an Alcoholics Anonymous session" (Miller 2004). Modeled on Twelve Step programs, drug courts preach the mantra of accepting personal responsibility for one's choices and the dangers of blaming others or of trying to change society. "The drug court's therapeutic paradigm requires the judge to discount the offenders' accounts of their goals for or responses to treatment unless they fit a fairly rigid script" (Miller 2004). Run fully at the discretion of the individual judge, each court sets its own schedule regarding how often offenders are required to come in (weekly, biweekly) and what tasks they are required to carry out. Often, judges require that participants go for regular drug testing, attend job-training programs, take medication prescribed by doctors, and participate in therapeutic groups. While the language used in drugs courts tends to emphasize treatment and "making the right choices," it is the power of the judge—as opposed to the lesser powers of probation officers, parole officers, and the like—that is seen as having the weight necessary to persuade drug addicts to change their ways.

In an era when social service budgets have dwindled and eligibility requirements for obtaining services have multiplied, drug courts have the resources to help participants gain access to health care, job training, and housing assistance that may otherwise entail very long waiting lists. In return for that largesse, however, the drug courts require participants to abide by the rules of other programs on the institutional circuit, and can punish participants for noncompliance (punishments include extending the drug court term and incarceration). While drug courts are often seen as a kinder and more therapeutic alternative to incarceration, the power of the drug court judge far exceeds that of the judge in traditional courtrooms, as new sanctions are regularly applied to defendants in drug courts with little possibility for due process. "The court, then, becomes concerned with behaviors that are not necessarily illegal but that courts stake their claim over in the name of recovery" (Brook 2010, p. 174).

Andrea, an African American woman in her forties, attended months of drug court sessions. "They [the judge] want me to see a psychiatrist. I go to all kinds of [AA and NA] meetings. I need them to sign. The judge is on my case." Neither a drug user nor a drug dealer (she was arrested because a relative sold drugs out of her apartment), Andrea eventually learned that her insistence that she was not an addict actually impeded her graduation from drug court. Once she picked up the language of affirming responsibility for one's choices, she was declared a "success." At the graduation ceremony she and the other graduates announced in a courtroom before their families, a judge, and various local dignitaries that they had formerly made bad choices and now had learned how to make good choices. (In the five-plus years we have known Andrea, we have never heard her spontaneously make similar remarks.) The graduates were congratulated, handed certificates, and sent on their way. Andrea, like many in her cohort, returned to the homeless shelter where she had been staying for the past year.

———

Given the Christian origins and ethos of AA/NA, its presence in the U.S. correctional system appears to contradict the First Amendment separation of church and state, yet it is rarely challenged in court.[7] In fact, collaborations between church and state have characterized moral crusades in the past, most notably during Prohibition, and American religious organizations and sentiments continue to influence public policy in matters such as abortion and marriage rights. More broadly, nation-states since the early modern period have worked in tandem with religious groups that train moral and faithful citizens and acknowledge the supremacy of the state (Sullivan 2009).

Examining emerging trends in U.S. constitutional law, Winnifred Sullivan (2010) observes that the courts increasingly interpret religion to be a natural, universal human need and thus a legitimate part of the responsibilities of the government to its citizens. Paradoxically, this judicial trend has developed at the same time as economic policies and rhetoric have increasingly cast suffering in terms of individual flaws and reduced the responsibility of the state for the well-being of its citizens (Crawford 2006). Deregulation of industry, lifetime limits on eligibility for public assistance under PRWORA, and privatization of government services (including prisons), to take but three examples, seem inconsistent with the expanded legal understanding of religion as a service that a responsive government legitimately provides its citizens. AA/NA offers a convenient way of resolving this tension. The claim that it is not a "religion" but is rather "spiritual" (a well-known AA/NA line being "Your Higher Power doesn't have to be God; it can be whatever you choose, even that chair over there") takes care of the First Amendment problem. And a moral platform of individual responsibility for one's problems, plus a plethora of volunteers who provide services free of cost to the state, takes care of the "big government" problem.

RELIGION OF INDIVIDUAL RESPONSIBILITY

Reflecting Boston's demographics, most of the study women grew up in Catholic families and christened their babies in Catholic churches. By the time they reached young adulthood, most had become disenchanted with Catholic churches that seemed out of touch with the harsh reality of their lives. Their negative feelings were confirmed when news of clergy sexual abuse dominated the Boston newspapers. For some, this corroborated what they already knew had been going on in churches for years; for others, the worst part of the revelations was the disproportionate attention paid to boys who had been molested, when girls are substantially more likely than boys to be targets of abuse. At this writing, the women tend to have more contact with the various Protestant churches that reach out to homeless and incarcerated populations. Typically, women's flirtations with these churches last for a few months or for as long as the church provides material support and a palpably warm welcome (cf. Crawford Sullivan 2011).

In contrast to their erratic church attendance, virtually all of the women tell us that spirituality is always important to them and that they deeply believe in God (cf. Crawford Sullivan 2011). Typically, the ways in which they talk about God reiterate the Twelve Step script, which, as we have argued, echoes the deeply rooted American ethos of individual choice. Elizabeth explained that God gives her choices but that she makes the wrong ones. Once, when Elizabeth had spoken at some length about God's presence in her life, we asked her why God gives her so much suffering. "It's not God's fault. When I drink, I don't take my meds." Echoing normative American morality, Elizabeth explains, "I believe God helps those who help themselves. I think God is giving me a test right now, which I probably deserve because there have been times I haven't appreciated what I had or done the right thing. But maybe I'm being hard on myself." Rounding out the theological landscape, after each stint in "recovery," Francesca reiterates that the solution to her problems of homelessness, abusive men, and chronic pain is "to turn it all over to God." Indeed, the very day that we drafted this chapter, she posted on Facebook: "I know that my life is unfolding according to your plan. Please send the wisdom and courage to accept that. Thanks, Me." And Carly, the youngest project participant, shares on Facebook ideas and aphorisms sprinkled with themes of surrender and powerlessness: "IF GOD COULD CHANGE ME HE CAN CHANGE ANYBODY AND ONCE U [sic] MAKE THE DECISION TO FOLLOW HIM AND TRUST HIM WITH YOUR LIFE AND SURRENDER TO HIM YOU WILL FEEL A HAPPINESS AND PEACE THAT NOTHING IN THIS WORLD CAN COMPARE TO."

It is not our intention to argue that religion necessarily contributes to the anguish experienced by poor and marginalized women. To the contrary, religious ideologies and leadership have inspired many oppressed people to come together and fight for freedom. In the United States the Catholic Workers Movement and the religiously driven civil rights ministry of the Reverend Dr. Martin Luther King, Jr. are particularly prominent examples. We also note the freedom that the Shakers afforded women in the nineteenth century and the vision of a nonpatriarchal cosmos imagined by Starhawk and other visionaries of the feminist spirituality movement (Sered 1994). Our argument is far more specific: the churches in which the women of this project were raised and the churches that most assertively reach out to them, as well as the Twelve Step groups and the quasi-religious institutions and organizations that provide services on the institutional circuit, preach the message, in one form or another, that pain and affliction are the consequences of one's individual choices and that neither social policies nor God should be blamed for allowing one to suffer.

CHAPTER 7

"Suffer the Children"

Fostering the Caste of the Ill and Afflicted

I will greatly multiply thy sorrow and thy conception; in sorrow thou shalt bring forth children.

—Genesis 3:16 (New American Standard Bible)

The christening was a festive event at the local Catholic church. Kahtia and Enrique were dressed to the nines, and Baby Sofie peeked out from the lace and tulle of her christening gown. The extended family of twenty or so buzzed with excitement when the priest called the parents up to the altar. Despite a couple of small glitches because Enrique couldn't quite understand what the priest asked him in English, the sense of joy was palpable when the baby was officially recognized as a child of God. While no one doubted Kahtia's maternity—she was enormous throughout the pregnancy—the status of Enrique's paternity was a bit murkier. Baby Sofie was conceived when Kahtia was raped shortly before she and Enrique met. Enrique had been absent at the conception, as was, one might surmise, God.

After the ceremony our straggling group of adults and children walked back to Kahtia and Enrique's house for the celebration. In the spirit of miraculous events, all twenty of us managed to squeeze into the two-room apartment. Kahtia, embracing the role of family matriarch, had prepared a veritable feast in a kitchen barely the size of a closet. Rice, pork, beans, and homemade tortillas—enough for at least forty people. She had even made a tray of macaroni and cheese to suit Susan's vegetarian diet.

Both Kahtia and Enrique had come a long way to get to this point. For Enrique, the road had been geographic: he had quite literally walked to the

United States from Central America. Kahtia, born less than a mile from the church, had traveled an even longer road of abuse, violence, and incarceration.

———

Kahtia's earliest memories are of Sunday dinners at the home of her Irish maternal grandparents. The clan, including Kahtia's mother and older sister, would be seated around the family table; Kahtia and her younger brother would eat out in the hall. The older sister's father was white, but an African American man was father to the two younger children. It was made clear that their dark skin color was not welcome at the dinner table.

An under-the-radar heroin addict, Kahtia's mother supported her habit by shooting up Kahtia and her brother with drugs and receiving money from the men she invited to rape them. Kahtia remembers her father as a good but weak man; he was an alcoholic and did not live with his children. She also remembers being told she exhibited "unruly behavior," and because of that, she was removed from home and placed in a residential program for "problem kids." Child Welfare Services did not believe Kahtia's stories of abuse, and she was sent home on weekends, where the rapes continued. By the time she was ten, Kahtia decided that anywhere she went would be better than home, so she ran away.

Living on the streets as a very young girl, Kahtia encountered her first bit of good luck: a Puerto Rican gang adopted her. With pride, Kahtia recounts how the gang leader heard of her as "the girl who kept a razor blade hidden inside her mouth" in order to defend herself. To this day, she identifies as Puerto Rican and feels strongly that the protection and affection of the gang is what saved her life. After a few years on the streets and in and out of juvenile institutions, Kahtia launched what at the time seemed to her a glamorous career as a prostitute and drug dealer in up-scale New York City clubs. Shortly thereafter, however, "I became my own best customer and had to go to the streets to make money for drugs." Street-level prostitution was not so glamorous. She learned to become totally numb and dissociate herself from the situation during sex. She demonstrated this by tipping her head back, closing her eyes, and dropping her jaw open. "It was just . . . wait for him to finish and give me the money."

By her late teens Kahtia had graduated from juvenile therapeutic institutions to juvenile detention facilities, and by her twenties she was serving significant time for prostitution and drug dealing. Between stints of incarceration, Kahtia married. Like many women who experience abuse as children, she married an abusive man. The children she had with him were taken into Child Welfare Services custody. A number of years later she married a man who seemed "more civilized." That marriage ended when she caught him in bed with her sister. After that, "I didn't care. I'd given up on life."

It was after twenty years of the streets, detox, jail, and rehab programs that we first met Kahtia, during the chaos of clothing distribution day at the women's drop-in center. Without a place to store their belongings, homeless women are in near-constant need of donated clothing. "You look like one hot mama," Francesca yelled out. "You go girl!" With a great deal of her bosom and belly hanging out of a shirt several sizes too small, Kahtia had come to the center for maternity clothes. Although the pregnancy was the result of rape, Kahtia was thrilled to be expecting a child. "I believe God gave me a second opportunity to be a mom. . . . The Lord is watching me. Otherwise I wouldn't survive." She explained that about a year earlier she had made a decision to stop using drugs. In her late thirties, "I was done. You can only run for so long. I was running from myself. I didn't know who I was." She was determined to stay out of prison: "I don't want another day of people telling me what to do, when to eat, when to sleep, when to shit." Having lost custody of her older children, Kahtia declared that she was ready to do whatever it took to keep this child. And this time she had more resources to rely on. She had a caseworker, a psychiatrist, and the support of a job-training program for former offenders. Even more important, Kahtia declared, "I have my own determination, and knowing that my younger brother [who had died three months earlier of a crack overdose] is watching over me." Also on her side this time was Enrique, the first man she had ever been involved with who was not an addict, a criminal, or a "player." A kind man (if, Kahtia felt, a bit on the slow side), he had never had children and was happy to accept the child she was carrying as his own. "He is my backbone."

A few months later Kahtia overdosed on her psychiatric medication (Clonidine and Hydroxyzine). In a sad and tired voice she told us that she and Enrique were living in one bedroom of an apartment that they shared with several other people. The stress of the close quarters, she explained, had a lot to do with her desire to overdose. She also was feeling down because she had just found out that because she had moved out of a shelter and in with Enrique, she no longer was considered to be homeless and had been taken off the priority list for public housing. In that moment, she had a fleeting thought that if she were to die, she could be with her late brother. Despite the incident, the baby was fine. Relieved that her actions had not hurt the child, she began picking out names and even felt the baby nudging her with its little feet as if to encourage her to stay strong.

———

A few weeks before her autumn due date Kahtia's water broke, and she and Enrique went to the hospital, where the doctors induced labor. The birth went well but the baby was lethargic and had an erratic heartbeat. After what seemed to us a very long time (nearly two days), the doctors figured out that Kahtia's antidepressants were affecting the baby. Although we were furious that Kahtia's doctor had not warned her ahead of time that her medication could create problems, Kahtia appeared inspiringly calm during the baby's weeklong stay in the neo-natal intensive care unit. Fortunately, she was allowed to remain in the hospital with her baby. This gave her a bit of time to rest, recover, and learn how to care for the newborn.

When we visited Kahtia and Baby Sofie (named after Kahtia's caseworker) a few weeks later, Kahtia was in fine form. Still carrying some baby weight, Kahtia looked happy and well put together. The baby had recovered from the medication and Kahtia was relishing her duties as a mother and housewife. Kahtia had had two baby showers—one organized by her rehabilitation program and the other by her auntie (her late father's sister)—and had received all of the necessary baby equipment. She, Enrique, and the baby still shared that same one bedroom, but the crib was beautifully decorated with pink bumpers, an entire teddy bear family, and a hand-knit blanket. Before long, Kahtia was up and about with the baby, going to all of her meetings, group sessions, and appointments. Her uncle and auntie came by daily to help with support and advice, and Enrique proposed marriage by surprising her with a ring inside a fortune cookie.

Over the next few months Kahtia, Enrique, and Sofie continued to thrive, but their living situation was becoming increasingly problematic. One of their roommates "picks on Enrique and he doesn't have the balls to stand up to him." Even worse, another one of the roommates had made a sexual advance on her. We talked about the possibility of reporting the incidents to the Boston Housing Authority to see if the family could be moved up on the priority list for public housing, but Kahtia pointed out that a report could backfire, possibly giving Child Welfare Services the ammunition to take Sofie from her. Her fears were not unfounded. Approximately half of the states in the United States list a caregiver's inability to provide shelter as justification for removing a child from its parents (Culhane et al. 2003).

––––––––

One warm spring day we met Kahtia at her apartment. In a low-cut caftan dress with spaghetti straps and an open back, her voluptuous cleavage was very much in evidence, and we spotted a new tattoo with Sofie's name on her left breast. We teased her, saying that she looked like a Puerto Rican mother of ten kids and twenty grandchildren. She laughed, liking this image for herself. She told us that she cleans and cooks every day for friends, family, and "homeless people," and very much enjoys being the family matriarch. When we walked with her to the grocery store, she seemed to know everyone in town, stopping every few steps to chat or give a cigarette to acquaintances too broke to buy their own.

During that period, whenever we visited Kahtia at her apartment or ran into her at a program, Sofie was with her, and she was always well groomed and fed, playing with appropriate toys for her age, and surrounded with love. Beneath the idyllic maternal surface, however, Kahtia struggled with her health. Her asthma had sent her to the emergency room. Her migraines were debilitating. Arthritis crept into all of her joints, and she hurt her back when she fell while washing the floor. In the wake of these setbacks, Kahtia had become anxious, agitated, and depressed. Feeling as if she was falling apart, the familiar cravings for drugs began to haunt her. With her anxiety flaring, she had asked her psychiatrist to put her on Klonopin (an anti-anxiety medication of the benzodiazepine group). He refused, telling her that she would probably become addicted. In the meantime she bounced from medication to medication as her psychiatrist tried to find something else that would work. "I'm not your rat lab," she retorted once in frustration. When the anxiety became unmanageable, she bought benzodiazepines from a friend.

By early summer, Kahtia was pregnant again, and Enrique was "ecstatic" that this would be his biological child. But when a genetic counselor recommended Kahtia have an abortion because the baby could have Down syndrome, Kahtia sank into suicidal ideations and almost wound up returning to the hospital. In the nick of time, her auntie came by the apartment to calm her down. Kahtia explained to us that she was not upset at the prospect of having a child with Down syndrome. Quite the opposite: she felt ready to welcome whatever child God sent her. Rather, it was being told she should have an abortion that caused the distress, perhaps because of her Catholic upbringing, or her own childhood experiences of being unwanted, or the loss of her older children, or perhaps because of all three. In any case, Kahtia feels strongly that every child deserves a chance to be loved. On more than one occasion Kahtia has voiced the idea that "the Lord is watching me. Otherwise I wouldn't survive. I've been gang-raped and beaten beyond recognition. . . . I believe God gave me a second opportunity to be a mom. . . . God didn't want me to get hurt, but he wanted me to be a mom."

In late summer Kahtia was informed that she would be moved to the highest priority for housing, but before she even had a chance to celebrate, she received a second letter telling her that because of her criminal record she was no longer eligible for public housing. Eight months pregnant and toting toddler Sofie through the sweltering city heat, she scrambled to acquire all kinds of certification and letters to prove to the Boston Housing Authority that she was sufficiently reformed and was no longer a risky tenant.

Baby Liliana was born healthy—no Down syndrome, and just as cute as her sister. But it was hard for Kahtia to relax with the new infant because of her financial worries. Her Child Welfare Services caseworker knew that Enrique was living with her (from the caseworker's perspective, this was a good thing as he is the baby's father), but the welfare office cut back her TANF remittance because, as the father, Enrique was expected to contribute money to the household. Enrique's erratic income as a gardener and mason, however, was not enough to keep them afloat. One day when we spoke on the phone, Kahtia was in tears: she had run out of formula for the baby and had no money to buy more.

One night Kahtia and Enrique had an argument. He was drinking, so she left the house. In a stroke of bad luck she ran right into a policeman who knew her from her street days. This particular officer, according to Kahtia, had told other people in the neighborhood that he was out to get her. (Kahtia did not explain why he was out to get her. On other occasions she told us that when she worked in prostitution, police officers often demanded sex from her.) Although he initially came to their apartment because of Enrique's drunken arguing, he ended up handcuffing Kahtia in front of her girls. After a night in jail she was charged with prostitution and given an August court date. She considered pleading guilty so that she could get it over with and not drag Sofie and Liliana through a trial. (Ultimately she decided against a guilty plea.) "I am on the road to a nervous breakdown because of Enrique, DSS [the Department of Social

Services; that is, Child Welfare Services], housing, and I'm about to run out of my meds. The psychiatrist isn't there anymore—I've seen three different psychiatrists in the last month—all at the same clinic. My meds are not working and I can't sleep." Making matters worse, she needed to recertify her SSI eligibility, but in order to do so, she needed a letter from her psychiatrist. However, because she had been assigned at least three different psychiatrists over the past six months, there was a delay in having the appropriate letter written for her. "I'm thinking of going back to the streets to get money the way I know how [prostitution]. . . . My babies are my life," Kahtia explained; "I will do whatever I need to do for them."

A few months later Kahtia was raped when she went out to deposit her Social Security check in the bank. (Several other women, including Elizabeth, told us that being assaulted on the day that Social Security or welfare checks arrive is quite common.) The attacker kicked her in the back of her neck and lower back, and choked her until she fell unconscious. All of her things were stolen—her phone, iPod, public-transportation pass, and money. Based on her description of the man who raped her, the police said that "he sounded like a man who has been doing this to working girls around here." They did not seem to be making much of an effort to find him. In the weeks following the rape, Kahtia felt renewed urges to use heroin; she spent many hours each day in tears and even considered suicide. She became afraid to go out of the house and stopped going to her various appointments and programs. Unable to deal with either the rape or Kahtia's reaction to it, Enrique moved out. When we stopped by to visit, she was in bad shape. Her hair looked stringy and unwashed. She was wearing an oversized man's T-shirt and a ripped skirt. For the first time since we had met her, the place was a mess, and she had sent her girls to stay for a few days with her cousin (a devout Christian with seven children of her own). At Kahtia's request we called her Child Welfare Services caseworker to report the rape. The caseworker—a twenty-year-old social work student—sounded totally out of her league concerning Kahtia. Positive that Enrique was the better parent, the caseworker told us that she was "sure" that Child Welfare Services would take the children from Kahtia.

THE MYTH OF THE BAD MOTHER

Mothers everywhere bear the impossible expectation that they can protect their children from the barbs of an outside world over which mothers have little control. While mothers around the world suffer from social assignments of responsibility for their children without the resources and authority to carry out those responsibilities in a satisfying way,[1] criminalized, poor, and other marginalized women experience extra doses of high responsibility and low authority. As a society, we blame and even punish "bad" mothers as individual deviants, regardless of the social conditions that make it difficult for many women to be "good" mothers. Dominant ideals of good mothering become an additional source of pain and injury for women who cannot afford the nice clothes, nutritious food, and the after-school clubs and activities that television families enjoy. As mothers, women are held responsible for their children's welfare in communities where keeping children safe is no small task, even while their authority as mothers is constrained not only by economic, racial, and gender inequalities but directly and explicitly by Child Welfare Services and the courts. Contemporary models of good mothers assume a fairly high income, a stable two-parent household, "and significant control over one's own destiny" (Connolly 2000, p. xvii). Bad mothers are disproportionately poor women and women of color whose parenting is more visible to government and public agencies than that of their white and middle-class counterparts. Low-income women are scrutinized by the government in Medicaid offices, public hospitals and clinics, welfare offices, and public housing and Section VIII inspections. Middle-class mothers may also abuse alcohol or prescription painkillers, but "bad mothers are the mothers who get caught" (Appell 1998, p. 357).

Kahtia does not fit popular dichotomies in which motherhood is idealized (mother as giver of unconditional love and nurture) or demonized ("unfit mother," "unnatural mother," "crack mother," or "monster mother"; cf. Connolly 2000; Humphries 1999). Like most mothers everywhere, Kahtia strongly embraces normative cultural ideologies of good mothering. She endeavors to enact those ideologies in her daily life; she is judged in light of those ideologies; and she interprets her own actions as those of a good mother. Mothering is central to her thoughts, feelings, conversations, choices, strategizing, actions, and self-presentation. She beams with pride at her daughters' accomplishments, stays up at night with them when they are sick, regularly puts her children's needs before her own, and tries her very best to raise children in difficult circumstances. Some of Kahtia's friends and acquaintances have ended up in jail for attempting to protect their children from abuse or for stealing in order to feed and house their children (cf. Ferraro & Moe 2003). Even while incarcerated, these women work to parent from a distance by arranging care with relatives, keeping on top of Child Welfare Services regarding appropriate placements, setting up visitation, checking to see if children are doing their homework and if they have been taken to the doctor for checkups, and trying to prearrange adequate housing for the family once they are released. Permanent loss of custody while in prison, in contrast, sets women up, in Kahtia's words, "to hit the streets running"—looking for drugs—when they are released.

Most of the women we have come to know over the past five years fluctuated between actively raising their children and temporarily or permanently losing custody. These personal vacillations are reflections of public policies that sometimes punish women for "poor mothering" and at other times give mothers special support and priority in terms of housing and other services. In the United States, mothering increasingly has become a target of legislative policy and judicial control. Abortion restrictions, prosecution of women for prenatal harm, TANF regulations regarding the spacing of children, removal of children from mothers who use drugs, policies that pit the rights of mothers against socially constructed notions of the "best interest of the child," contract motherhood (so-called surrogacy), and the authority of family courts in child custody decisions are all manifestations of a broad cultural consensus that the state can and should determine what constitutes good mothering and decide which mothers are good or bad.

KAHTIA

With the prostitution case hanging over her head and the sense that at any minute she could be picked up and incarcerated for probation violation, Kahtia decided it would be best for her to turn herself in and wrap up her sentence. By Kahtia's calculation, if she were to go to jail, she would be sent to a prerelease program (like the halfway house where we initially met many of the project women) in a few months, and then at her court date (which happened to be scheduled for her late brother's birthday, which she saw as an indication that he was watching over her), she'd be sent home to finish off a few months' parole. In short, she just wanted to finish dealing with the correctional system for good. In the meantime, Enrique would move back in and take care of the girls.

———

The Suffolk County House of Corrections, located near Boston's homeless shelters, soup kitchens, and public hospital, is a stark, multistory building tucked away on a street with no parking, either on the street or in public lots. We sat down with Kahtia in a brightly decorated playroom usually reserved for incarcerated mothers visiting with their children. After greeting and catching up on our lives, she told us that she quite liked her mental health worker in jail. However, there had been delays in her seeing a psychiatrist to get her medication straightened out. She was finally prescribed Celexa (an antidepressant), but was given nothing for her anxiety and panic attacks. She was also attending numerous classes and programs: Health and Realization (she liked this one, a self-help group in which "I learn to listen to myself"), Art and Spirituality, Relapse Prevention, Freedom from Violence, and AA. While she enjoyed and was learning from the programs, she was also well aware that the programs give certificates that would look good when the time came to request a prerelease placement and try to get into public housing. Her one request of us was to bring her a copy of *The Diary of Anne Frank*.

Shortly after our visit, Kahtia's auntie died. This was a terrible loss for Kahtia and her daughters, the most immediate consequence of which was that now there was no longer a person designated by the prison to bring Kahtia's children to visit her. Enrique was not allowed in, because he was an undocumented immigrant. Because Kahtia had not lost custody of the girls, Child Welfare Services claimed that it was not its responsibility to bring the girls to see her. Together with Kahtia we spent many hours writing letters and making phone calls trying to arrange authorization for us to bring the girls to visit, but to no avail. After two months without personal contact, her relationship with her girls deteriorated. Her older daughter, now almost three years old, refused to speak to her on the phone, and Kahtia became increasingly depressed and anxious. Following months of "making progress" (her therapist's words), Kahtia attempted suicide three months before the end of her sentence, was put in solitary confinement to "calm down," and was denied the early release that previously had seemed likely.

COLLATERAL CAPTIVES

Approximately 70 percent of American women under correctional control in prison or on probation or parole are mothers of minor children; 15 percent have infants under six weeks old; between 5 and 10 percent enter correctional facilities while pregnant; and more than half of mothers in state prisons reported living with at least one of their children in the month before their arrest (Arriola, Braithwaite, & Newkirk 2006; Travis & Waul 2003; Glaze & Maruschak 2010). Currently, the parents of one in every fifty children in the United States are in prison (Phillips 2013).

The children of parents who have been incarcerated are more likely than other children to become lifelong members of the caste of the ill and afflicted, and all the evidence points to the size of that caste increasing over the following decades (cf. Phillips et al. 2006). When mothers are sent to prison, their children become collateral captives, following their mothers into the institutional circuit and often ending up in foster care or living with an extended family member who may be less able to parent than the incarcerated mother was. While many foster families take in children for all of the best reasons, other foster care settings seem to set children up for lifelong problems. Foster children are prescribed cocktails of powerful antipsychotic drugs just as frequently as the most mentally disabled children, if not more frequently, and at twice the rate of children not in the foster care system. Risperdal, Seroquel, and other drugs that were developed for schizophrenia are prescribed regularly even though schizophrenia is extremely rare in children. According to the Government Accountability Office (2012), children in foster care are prescribed psychotropic drugs at higher levels than considered safe by the Food and Drug Administration. Even children under one year old have been prescribed these drugs, many of which have side-effects of drowsiness and rapid weight gain and carry the risk of creating metabolic problems. In what Dr. Paula Rochon (Rochon & Gurwitz 1997) has termed a "prescribing cascade," doctors prescribe still other drugs to manage the side-effects (Zito et al. 2008).

As had been the case for Kahtia herself, children who spend time in foster or institutional care are disproportionately likely to later spend time in juvenile detention centers. "The assumption of pathologies lies at the heart of [the juvenile detention center], and rationalizes how the children are treated, caged and punished" (Bickel 2010). In a study of 100,000 juvenile offenders from an urban county over a period of ten years, Anna Aizer and Joseph J. Doyle Jr. (2011) found a much greater likelihood of adult incarceration (approximately three times higher) for those incarcerated as juveniles compared to juveniles who committed the same crimes but were not incarcerated. The same study found the impact of juvenile incarceration on rates of adult incarceration to be even greater for girls than for boys.

For Katia, as for most incarcerated mothers, separation from their children compounds their punishment and their suffering and losses. Throughout her sentence Kahtia counted the days until reunification with her daughters, convincing herself that everything would be wonderful once she could be with her children. But the post-incarceration reality for mothers is far from easy. In prison women may fantasize about being perfect mothers to angelically behaved children, but find upon release they are not perfect and that their children are not angels. Rather, relationships need to be renegotiated with children who may be angry that their mothers left and afraid that their mothers will leave again. Mothers may be surprised at how much their children have grown and changed. Mothers may feel overwhelmed upon moving from a prison setting in which everything is decided for you to a home setting where you are responsible not only for all of your own needs and decisions but also for those of your children. Especially mothers who lack economic resources may struggle to give their children all that they had hoped they could, while also trying to get their own lives back together (cf. Flores & Pellico 2011).

KAHTIA

Upon leaving prison, Kahtia asked the Department of Transitional Assistance (or DTA, the state welfare agency) to help her get into a family shelter with her daughters. She and the girls were sent to what is called a scatter shelter in a town located forty-five minutes of highway driving away from Boston. Kahtia was told that this would be an intermediate stage to getting into a real family shelter with support services and appropriate accommodations for children. The scatter shelter was actually an Extended Stay America hotel on the side of a highway with no accessible public transportation. Moving there required her to take her daughters out of their preschool in Boston. There was no play space or activities for the many children staying at the shelter; mothers and children were essentially cooped up in hotel rooms twenty-four hours a day.

At first, what was hardest for Kahtia was the uncertainty. No one told her how long she would be there—a few days, a few weeks, or longer. We spoke to her caseworker, who sternly told us to make sure Kahtia understood that if she left this scatter shelter, she could not reapply for help from the DTA for one full year. The caseworker was not able to give any estimate of how long

Kahtia would be there. Her only advice was that Kahtia appeal on the basis of the Americans with Disabilities Act that because of her mental health disability she needed to be closer to her therapist and doctor. But even so, the caseworker told us, it could be months before the family would be placed in a family shelter closer to Boston.

After six months the scatter shelter was taking a toll on Kahtia and the girls. She couldn't get to church, the supermarket, or a meeting with her therapist, because she had no means of transportation. The only store within walking distance was a convenience store that did not accept vouchers from WIC (the federal program that provides certain free food to pregnant women and young children). Kahtia had to pay over $6 to get juice for the girls that would have free through WIC. Then, because she was living in a shelter and not paying rent, her SSI was reduced. The move into the shelter also reduced her welfare and food stamp resources (the latter most likely because of a bureaucratic error). At one point, she resorted to prostitution to get money to buy food for her children.

Impressed with Kahtia's mothering, her Child Welfare Services worker offered to begin the process of closing the case on the girls (that is, releasing Kahtia and Enrique from government supervision) but insisted that Kahtia come into Boston for weekly urine tests. Kahtia went twice (both tests were clean), but the transportation cost was out of reach. On top of the expense of the cab ride to get to the bus that took her to the train that connected to another bus, the trip took two hours. Not only did she have her own transportation costs to worry about, but there were those of her daughters too. At one point Liliana developed a pus-filled lump the size of a golf ball on her back. Kahtia called an ambulance, and mother and daughter were taken to a local hospital. There she was told Liliana needed surgery, and the staff sent her to a larger Boston hospital. Because the infection turned out to be multi-drug-resistant *Staphylococcus aureus* (MRSA) and did not heal well, Kahtia was instructed to bring Liliana to the local pediatrician for daily appointments. The taxi rides cost $20 each way. Echoing Francesca's words, Kahtia—in tears—told us that no matter how hard she tries, she just can't seem to catch a break.

After months of misery in the scatter shelter, Kahtia came up with the idea of writing to Massachusetts governor Deval Patrick. His "housing person" got in touch with her, and within a few weeks Kahtia and her daughters were moved to a much better equipped family shelter in Boston. Kahtia put the girls back in preschool, where Sofie attended a bilingual class and proudly taught Kahtia and Enrique "The Itsy Bitsy Spider" song in Spanish. Child Welfare Services indicated that Kahtia had proven herself a responsible parent and that the agency was closing her case. However, this meant that Child Welfare Services would no longer pay for her children to attend or be transported to preschool. Kahtia knew the girls were better off in preschool than sitting in a room in the shelter all day, so when it came down to the last two weeks of urine testing required by Child Welfare Services, she skipped a week so that the case would not be closed.

All in all, things were now much better for Kahtia and the family. Three days a week she attended a day program for people with dual diagnoses (mental illness and substance abuse). The program consisted of groups such as art therapy and journal writing. She was assigned a new psychiatrist and put on nine medications—five psychiatric and four others, including one for pain. When we asked her what meds she was taking, she laughed because there were so many. The only ones she could remember were Thorazine, Neurontin, Hydroxychloroquine (for arthritis), and Protazen (an antidepressant/anxiety suppressor).

Throughout this period Kahtia and Enrique held long conversations during which they decided that they were both committed to being a family. On an early summer day they were married in a modest ceremony at City Hall. Kahtia dressed up in a lovely long off-white gown and glittery, skyscraper-high-heeled shoes that Enrique had picked out at a local shop. Enrique looked smart in a tan suit, and the girls wore adorable matching pink frilly outfits. The entire ceremony took less than five minutes, but having already waited for two hours out in the hall due to some unexplained bureaucratic delay, the girls were tired, cranky, and clingy during the ceremony. The justice of the peace did not bother pronouncing Kahtia's name properly (he called her Kathryn), and Enrique suddenly forgot his English.

———————

The next winter we went for a walk around the neighborhood with Kahtia while the girls were in preschool. Usually conversational and engaging, that day Kahtia had her eyes glued to the cell phone she held in her palm. Noticing our questioning looks, she explained, "I have an app on my phone that takes your address and shows you where registered sex offenders live in your vicinity. Look at this map. There are fifteen predators right in this neighborhood, and my angels, my babies are here. I walk down the street and I look for them. It's an obsession," she said. "It's not healthy to be doing this." We asked her if any of the men who have hurt her have ever been punished. "No," she replied, as she fumbled in her pocketbook for a bottle of anti-anxiety pills that she had purchased from a friend.

CHAPTER 8

Gender, Drugs, and Jail

"A System Designed for Us to Fail"

By the end of the first decade of the twenty-first century, approximately one in 89 American women was under correctional control in prison or on probation or parole.
—Pew Charitable Trusts, "One in 31: The Long Reach of American Corrections" (2009)

When the United States embarked on a policy that might well be described as mass incarceration, few considered the impact that this correctional course change would have on women.
—Meda Chesney-Lind, "Imprisoning Women: The Unintended Victims of Mass Imprisonment" (2002)

MCI-Framingham, the only Massachusetts state prison for women, is not an easy place to visit. The closest mode of public transportation lets passengers off more than a mile away from the prison. Trains to and from Boston run three times daily; the last train leaves Framingham at 2 P.M. Since visiting hours are from 1 P.M. to 4 P.M. and from 5 P.M. to 8:45 P.M., anyone coming to visit a mother, daughter, sister, or friend at MCI-Framingham must have a car or a couple hundred dollars to pay for taxis. Most incarcerated women come from poor families, and many women do not see their children or families for months at a time while at MCI.

We were lucky—we had a car. Following signs past the industrial outskirts of the city of Framingham, we drove up to a large fenced complex with— ironically—ample parking for visitors. We walked through the parking lot up to the main prison entrance, where we followed signs to the registration desk. Earlier, when we had called ahead to ask about visiting the prison, we were told that we should not bring anything in with us other than a state-issued ID. But after a lengthy wait in the check-in line, we learned that we would need to leave our coats and car keys in a locker for which we would need quarters to open the lock. After going back to the car for the quarters, back to the prison, and back in line, we signed up to visit Isabella and received a locker and visitor's pass. Then we sat down to wait—and wait and wait. For us this was not too arduous. For small children eager to see their mothers the two-hour or longer wait was much harder. Finally, we were called to the security desk, searched, stamped on the hand, and put on an elevator.

A stark and colorless space, the visitor's room was set up with chairs for visitors placed in a large circle facing inward. We were directed to sit in the one unoccupied seat. Then Isabella was called into the room and sent to a stacked pile of chairs in the corner from which she picked one up and brought it over to sit facing us in a second circle inside the larger circle. Signs around the room, plus frequent announcements by the guards, warned us that "physical contact between visitors and inmates shall be limited to a brief greeting at the start and at the completion of a visit. Excessive or inappropriate physical contact may be cause for termination of the visit and loss of privileges. Inmates are required to sit with their back flat against the chair and their feet flat on the ground. Legs may not be crossed and there is no straddling on the chairs."

We had trouble recognizing Isabella. Whereas she is typically very well groomed, today her hair looked stringy and dirty, her skin was blotchy, and her face had no makeup. In the prison-issue green T-shirt with "DOC" (Department of Corrections) stamped in large letters on the back, she looked eerily like the other forty or so inmates sitting in the interior circle facing their visitors. Normally bubbly and loquacious, Isabella was blank-faced and robotic, yawning and taciturn throughout what felt to us like an uncomfortable visit. After an awkward conversational pause we asked Isabella if there was anything we could do to help. She asked if we could put the equivalent of the monthly mass-transit pass project incentive in her prison account. With no source of money, she couldn't obtain items such as coffee, shampoo, and postage stamps that prisoners must purchase out of their own funds at the canteen, where most items are sold at substantially above-market prices. While we exchanged a few more desultory bits of information, guards circulated around the room, stopping here and there to listen to conversations. We, too, could easily hear the conversations taking place on either side of us.

Several months later, after she was released, we asked Isabella what had been going on when we visited. She explained that during the first month in prison she was detoxing from methadone, which is not used in prison. "Methadone detox is the worst detox because methadone is stored in the bone marrow. It's painful and scary and takes a very long time. You can't sleep for weeks. They don't give any medication for comfort here. . . . I was just left to detox on my own. It was terrible." Also, she explained, she'd had some serious "losing it" episodes while detoxing and, as a result, had spent quite a bit of time in the "hole" (solitary confinement).

ISABELLA'S PATH TO PRISON

For nearly all of the five-plus years we have known her, Isabella has looked and sounded like the educated, thirty-something soccer mom that in her heart she knows herself to be. Raised in an upper-middle-class white suburb, Isabella grew up believing that she would attend college, work for a few years, marry, and then raise a family of her own. In her community, sexual abuse was not on the radar, which is why, Isabella supposes, no one noticed that a "so-called family friend molested me as long as I remember—until I started running away when I was twelve." When Isabella was seventeen, she became pregnant. In her Catholic family, abortion was not an option. Though a consistently straight-A student, Isabella began to be treated as a pariah in her elite parochial school and was barred from social and extracurricular activities. The principal insisted that Isabella return to school two weeks after the baby was born. With no accommodations that would allow her to care for her daughter during the day, she had to leave the child with her mother, who eventually won custody of the child.

Like nearly one-third of American women today, Isabella gave birth by cesarean section.[1] In her case, the obstetrician selected by her parents prescribed Oxycontin for the post-surgical pain. After several weeks, when the doctor wouldn't give her more pills, she began to buy them from friends. "I didn't realize I was addicted for quite a while," Isabella recalls. She managed to graduate from high school and even made it through a few years of college before the cycle of drug use (including heroin), therapy, rehab, Alcoholics Anonymous, relapse, petty crime, and jail time became the borders of her life. Over the years Isabella has been raped, beaten up, locked up, and put down. She suffers from ulcers, anxiety, panic attacks, and night terrors so severe that she sometimes chooses to sleep with a man she does not care for just so she will not be alone when she wakes up screaming in the middle of the night. Most painful of all, she has been deprived of a relationship with her daughter.

In every conversation that we have had with Isabella, she has spoken about her daughter—how proud she is of her daughter's accomplishments in school and how much it hurts not to be able to be with her when Isabella is incarcerated or when her parents, who have custody, do not allow her to visit. For a period of time Isabella had to pay $50 an hour plus gas mileage for a court-appointed supervisor whenever she wanted to take her daughter out for a meal or shopping trip, regardless of the fact that she has never been suspected or accused of child neglect or endangerment. While her parents have permitted Isabella from time to time to be involved in her daughter's life—for example, Isabella was allowed to help her daughter choose her dress and get ready for her junior prom—her parents have also insisted on hair analyses to prove that Isabella has not used drugs. At $180 a pop, these tests are out of reach on Isabella's minimum-wage salary. Isabella's parents refuse to tell her daughter where Isabella has gone when she is away in rehabilitation or prison. Isabella's great fear is that her daughter will think that she has chosen to abandon her.

———————

A year or so after we first met Isabella, she reconnected with Reese, a lively woman with whom she had developed a romantic relationship during an earlier prison stay. Reese's cousin, who had taken custody of the children while Reese was in prison, was happy to return the kids to their mom and Isabella while custody arrangements were wending their way through the courts. Reese's two small children quickly began to call Isabella "Mummy Isabella," a role she embraced with all of her heart. The four of them moved into a small studio apartment with a yard where the kids could ride their tricycles. Life finally seemed good: Isabella was in a supportive and drug-free relationship, and she and Reese and the kids made a loving and warm family. "Reese and I are on the same level in terms of wanting the same things in life," Isabella told us. "And Reese has never been a drug user; that helps me in my ability to stay clean."

For several years things went well. Isabella and Reese both worked, and Isabella began paying off fines and court fees so that she could wrap all of her outstanding cases. Isabella and Reese shared the childcare, arranging their work schedules so that one of them always was home with the kids. Isabella adored the kids and the domesticity of her relationship with Reese. When we stopped by to visit, we'd find them socializing with other parents of young children, taking the kids to the playground, or cooking kid-friendly meals. "It's good being busy and having a purpose. The kids depend on us," Isabella said. Seeing how settled and sober Isabella had become, her mother was allowing her to see her daughter much more frequently. "My daughter and I are best friends. She tells me everything, asks my advice for everything; I love it." As the icing on the cake, her daughter was about to turn eighteen—at which point she and Isabella could not be prohibited from seeing one another or living together. Isabella allowed herself to hope that she and Reese could find a larger apartment with a room for her daughter.

Housing was very much on their minds. To regain legal custody of her children (who were already living with her), Reese needed to show Child Welfare Services that she had a three-bedroom apartment in which her son and daughter would each have his or her own room. Reese was approved for a state housing subsidy, so she and Isabella gave notice on their studio apartment and put down a deposit on a three-bedroom flat. However, before they could move, they were informed that the housing program's budget had been cut and Reese's subsidy had been reduced. Unable to find an apartment that they could afford and that met the requirements of Child Welfare Services, they moved in with Reese's family in an economically depressed central-Massachusetts town. Reese's mother, a "Jesus fanatic" (in Isabella's words), did not hide her dislike for Isabella's middle-class mannerisms or for Isabella and Reese's relationship. Isabella's ninety-minute commute to the restaurant job where she was on her feet fifty hours every week did not make things easier.

———

Isabella began to suffer excruciating migraine headaches. In addition, she had always been bothered by ulcers and reflux, but when she passed out at work one day and was rushed to the hospital, she was diagnosed with Crohn's disease. After several months Isabella gave up on continuing to live with Reese. She quit her job and then moved in with a male friend. A nice guy, Mark shared his bed with her.

She had been with Mark for a short while when, to her astonishment and delight, she found out that she was pregnant. This was the first time since her daughter was born that Isabella had been able to conceive. For the next three

months all Isabella could think or talk about was her engagement ring, ultra-
sounds, baby names, and maternity clothes. She was even more thrilled when
Reese and the kids moved into a nearby apartment. They arranged that Reese
would go back to work and Isabella would look after the kids. Mark's fourteen-
year-old son had always been living with his dad, and Isabella was ecstatic at
the prospect of mothering four children.

Seventeen weeks into the pregnancy Isabella went into early labor. She had
been passing large blood clots for several days and had gone to the emergency
room, where she was told nothing could be done about the condition and was
sent home. Waking up in the middle of the night in terrible pain, she went to
the bathroom and passed the baby. When Mark pulled it out of the toilet,
they saw the baby breathe and move. Then it died. The autopsy showed that
the baby had a hole in its heart and wouldn't have survived even if it had been
full term. Isabella was far along enough in the pregnancy for her breasts to
produce milk. For the next few weeks she cried and mourned, and then turned
back to heroin.

Things went from bad to worse. A neighbor knocked on their door in the
middle of the night looking for drugs. Mark went downstairs to tell her they
didn't have any. She bit him. When Isabella joined in the argument, the girl
bit her as well. Isabella shoved her, and she fell, opening a gash in her head.
Realizing that Isabella's criminal record was worse than his (Isabella was on
a "hold without bail" list), Mark told her to go back upstairs before the police
came so that he could take the charge for pushing the girl. Mark went to jail
and served a two-month sentence. Before he left, Isabella lobbied to keep his
son home with her, but Child Welfare Services decided that he should stay
with his grandmother in another town while his father was in jail. "Too many
children have been torn out of my arms," Isabella sobbed.

And then things went from worse to unthinkable. It turns out that the girl
with whom they fought is related to a "mafia rat" (Isabella's term) who arranged
for several of his buddies to break into Isabella and Mark's house and steal all
the electronics. With Mark still in jail, they raped Isabella, stole Mark's phone,
and texted her family members, telling them what they had done to Isabella.

With all of this going on, Isabella began to realize that she would not be
able to pull her life together as long as she still had open court cases. Despite
efforts to hold down a job, she still owed $12,000 in restitution fees from an
old charge of identity fraud left over from her drug-using days. As long as she
remained on probation, any interaction with police or courts (even a traffic

violation) carried the risk that she could be held without bail. "It's a system that is designed for us to fail," Isabella explains. People eagerly agree to long probations, for example, because they want to minimize jail time. But the probation conditions make it impossible for them to hold down jobs after they are released. They must come in for frequent urine tests and meetings with the parole officer, and they are required to attend numerous (sometimes daily) AA or NA meetings. "Employers are not interested in keeping employees who constantly are leaving work for these things," Isabella observed. "I hit the junkie ceiling—like the glass ceiling for women. I can't go further because of my record and probation conditions. I don't earn enough money for a decent life so I go back to using."

After a great deal of soul-searching and weighing of options, Isabella decided to tell the court that she would serve out the remaining six months of her sentence.[2] The jail term would substitute for her restitution fees, though the person she stole from will never get his money back. In addition, her incarceration would cost the Commonwealth of Massachusetts more than $200 per day.[3]

Isabella put her things in order, told her daughter that she would be going away for six months (she didn't tell her where), and went back to prison.

GENDER IN JAIL

In policy and practice, the correctional system reinforces the inequalities, violence, and miseries that set women up for incarceration. Women's prisons, more than men's prisons, impose myriad petty rules regarding hairstyles, neatness, and the like that seem intended to enforce normative gender roles (cf. Owen 1998). Ashley, a white woman in her mid-twenties explains, "In women's prisons male guards bust our asses on petty stuff. They don't do that in men's prisons, because they don't want to cause riots." "What kinds of petty things?" we asked. "You can't wear shower shoes in the day room. And there is a stricter dress code for women. Women can't wear white T-shirts because your bra outline shows. Women can't roll up their sleeves or their pants. Guards enforce the rule that beds are made by 7 A.M." Since there is little violence in women's prisons (at least in Massachusetts), these rules do not seem to be aimed at public safety or crowd control but rather at controlling the individual. This is made clear in the many prisons that keep women in shackles during labor and delivery (Center for Reproductive Rights 2010). As a twenty-one-year old African American prisoner who had been confined in a control unit (solitary confinement) told Cassandra Shaylor (1998, p. 392), "They don't do this because of 'safety and security of the institution,' they do it for humiliation."

The United States is one of the few countries in the world in which male correctional employees are permitted direct physical contact with female inmates and are employed to watch women shower, use the toilet, and give birth (A. Davis and Shaylor 2001). In Massachusetts these practices were halted in response to a well-publicized scandal in the 1990s (Rathbone 2007), but in other states male guards routinely pat down and search women prisoners. "Having male guards sends a message that female prisoners have no right to defend their bodies," explains former political prisoner Laura Whitehorn. Indeed, "putting women under men in authority makes the power imbalance as stark as it can be, and results in long-lasting repercussions post-release" (Whitehorn, quoted in Bader 2012a). Nationally, sexual abuse of women prisoners by male guards is so widespread that "it has been described as 'an institutionalized component of punishment behind prison walls'" (Buchanan 2007, p. 1). Because prisoners' grievances are filed internally, prison authorities can filter complaints (Buchanan 2007).

Revelations of widespread sexual abuse of women soldiers and cover-ups of that abuse in the United States military demonstrate that systems relying on the chain of command to pursue justice cannot be counted on to serve the needs of those who lack power within the institution. The impunity with which guards can rape women inmates is a consequence of the radical status disparities that are the foundation of prison culture. Women who might consider lodging a complaint don't, because, quite reasonably, they fear retaliation such as transfer to a prison far away from their family or being sent to the hole (solitary confinement). Government authorities, including prisons and jails, are immune from "vicarious liability," meaning that the sexual misconduct of a prison guard is not considered the fault of the prison as an institution unless the prisoner can prove that the guard's conduct resulted from a government policy, custom, or practice (Buchanan 2007). While rape involving physical force is not rampant in Massachusetts's women's prisons, it is quite common for male guards to use their status and power to coerce women to engage in sexual contact in return for, in Isabella's words, "things from the outside like cigarettes or even food." Sexual favors may be traded for minor privileges or even in return for such basic rights as permission to call one's children.

Beyond these obvious abuses of power, routine prison procedures such as requiring the removal of clothing, intimate touching of an inmate's body in strip searches and medical exams, use of shackles, and the threat or use of physical force are especially traumatizing for women with abuse histories (that is, the majority of incarcerated women). Women who have suffered past abuse are particularly sensitive to coercive situations. Responses to perceived threat include hypervigilance, interpersonal distrust, alienation, withdrawal, fighting back, extreme outbursts, worsening of psychiatric symptoms or physical health problems, self-injury or suicide attempts, and increased substance use (Veysey, Coue, & Prescott 1998; Haney 2003). In a prison context, such behaviors can lead to further punishment, including solitary confinement. Isabella's experiences were not unusual; most of the women of this project have spent at least some time in solitary. For Isabella, as for many other inmates, the lack of social connections during solitary confinement as well as the sensory deprivation and twenty-four-hour observation by guards exacerbated her fears and anxiety (cf. Shaylor 1998).

MEDICALIZATION, CRIMINALIZATION, AND THE MYTH OF CHOICE

We opened this book with the question: Have prisons become the way that America deals with human suffering? At this point we offer this answer: Not exclusively. Rather, prison is the ultimate station on a path that begins with a cultural consensus that the individual is responsible for his or her own misery, a path on which criminalization and medicalization are—all too often—a double-edged sword. The boundary between punishing and helping institution blurs when women attend the same Twelve Step–type programs and classes in both sets of institutions, see the same brands of therapists and psychiatrists in both sets of institutions, and are tested for "dirty urine" in both sets of institutions. Treatment and punishment merge when access to basic civil rights (such as a monthly SSI or SSDI remittance) depends on doctors' diagnoses. It is difficult to see much of a difference between "crime" and "disease" when, as in Massachusetts, 59 percent of incarcerated women are classified as "open mental health cases" and 49 percent are treated with psychiatric medication in prison (Massachusetts Department of Corrections 2013).[4] Numbers of this magnitude suggest either that some women are locked up for the "crime" of being mentally ill or that some incarcerated women are medicated when they are not mentally ill.[5]

Nationally, approximately 11 percent of male inmates, and approximately twice that proportion of women inmates, had an overnight hospital stay due to psychiatric problems before admission to prison (Sabol 2011). These numbers are in part a consequence of the lack of resources for community mental health services and long-term supportive housing, a shortfall that contributes to jails and prisons becoming the de facto mental health system for large numbers of Americans. In part, these numbers highlight the extent to which legal and illegal psychoactive medications are used to address the same kinds of problems. And, in part, these numbers reflect the broad social disapprobation both of mental illness and of illicit drug use.

Summarizing the literature on "transinstitutionalization" (mental hospitals to prisons), Melissa Thompson (2010) notes that women inmates are medicated at much higher rates than male inmates and are more likely to receive psychiatric evaluations than men even when they do not self-report mental illness. Studies show that receiving a psychiatric evaluation reduces the chances that a defendant will have the charges against him or her dropped. It also increases the likelihood of conviction, incarceration, and a lengthier sentence. While psychotropic medication can stabilize inmates who otherwise might be unable to work with their legal representatives, the *overuse* of psychotropic drugs can interfere with prisoners' ability to participate in the preparation of their defense. Functioning as "chemical restraints," psychotropic drugs may be used to restrict autonomy in much the same way as shackles and solitary confinement are used (Leonard 2002).

Some months after finishing the structured part of this project, we chatted with Isabella once again about her prison experiences. The next day she wrote us the following message, clarifying her understanding of the relationship between medicalization and criminalization:

> To explain where I came up with that, most of the women that I've been in Framingham with come in there addicted to SOMETHING. Normally its drugs n alcohol, [but] you'd be amazed at the addictive personalities I've seen in some of the women who are self-proclaimed "normal" (their way of saying they're non addicts, which I've also noticed is a double entendre for they are "better than" addicts) . . . so the women come in addicted, to whatever is their "poison," so to speak, which society sees as a problem, obviously [or] they wouldn't be in prison. Then the prison doctors prescribe the women a whole smorgasbord of medication that they may or may not need: I'm with the people who believe the meds are NOT NEEDED, mostly because depression and anxiety are signs of withdrawal. Those women who show signs of anxiety and depression who are NOT in withdrawals, at least not physically, are most likely depressed because they are in prison . . . same with the anxiety. But

here's where it gets sticky; you have almost 1,000 women in framingham on any given day, and if you took a close look at the medication lists, you would see the EXACT SAME PROTOCOL for almost every woman in medication. Now I'm no expert in medication, or a licensed prescriber, but that's gotta say something about the LACK of attention or care or even just the THOUGHT PROCESS before putting that pen to the prescription pad to the individual before them. Again, I'm no expert, but I'd bet dollars to donuts that the statistics on the actual medications prescribed to most of the women in MCI Framingham have to be tied to some deal with the pharmaceutical companies or something. They HAVE to be . . . because I've seen the changes in medications over the years . . . from one set list of the meds to another. First it was Seraquel, Effexor, Clonidine, and Trazedone for sleep. Now its Neurontin, Thorazine, Selexa, and Doxepin for sleep. It's almost like when you see in movies the guys that work for Phizer going to Drs. offices and giving them samples and then asking [the] Drs to push the new meds on their patients.

PRISON AND INEQUALITY

Rather than preventing or correcting problems, correctional system policies and culture replicate and intensify the inequalities and the structural violence that create and sustain the caste of the ill and afflicted. Mass incarceration is part of a larger landscape of racial inequality that concentrates poor schools, poor health, and poverty in segregated neighborhoods. Racism is reinscribed by laws mandating longer sentences for crack cocaine (more readily available in black communities) than powder cocaine (more readily available in white communities), and exacerbated when prison guards—disproportionately poor and poorly educated white men from rural backgrounds—are placed inside overcrowded prisons and tasked with controlling large populations disproportionately made up of people of color. Being poor increases one's chances of landing in prison, but a prison record permanently reduces one's chance of earning a decent salary or even landing a job. Prisons are used as a solution to the consequences of violence against women, but incarcerated women face abuse at the hands of prison guards while incarcerated men are immersed in cultures of prison violence. Prisons have come to be used as a solution for managing people deemed mentally ill, but prisons serve as breeding grounds for anxiety, depression, panic, and psychosis (Metzner & Fellner 2010). Often the residence of last resort for Americans suffering from chronic illness, prisons provide fertile environments for the spread of MRSA (antibiotic-resistant staph infection), tuberculosis, and other infectious diseases (National Commission on Correctional Health Care 2002; Mukherjee et al. 2013).

Like Isabella, women in Massachusetts are typically incarcerated for non-violent, drug-related crimes for which they serve sentences of one year or less. Many are locked up for probation or parole violation (such as missing meetings with parole officers, failing urine tests, dropping out of therapeutic or rehab programs, committing traffic violations) or for failure to pay restitution or court costs in the wake of offenses that initially were deemed too minor to warrant prison time. Nearly half of the women admitted annually to MCI-Framingham are awaiting trial; that is, *they have not been convicted or sentenced* (Massachusetts Department of Corrections 2013). For the most part, these women are being held because they cannot afford to pay bail, sometimes as low as $100 (Massachusetts Department of Corrections 2013). Although women constitute only 7 percent of state prisoners, they make up 33 percent of *pretrial* detainees held by the Massachusetts Department of Corrections. "There are lots of women in the Awaiting Trial Unit who are $10 short on bail," Isabella reported. "They can pay most of it but not all, so they are kept in jail, which costs the state a lot more." In fact, the average cost per year to house an inmate in a Massachusetts state prison is $47,102 (Massachusetts Executive Office of Public Safety and Security 2013).

The incarceration of low-income Americans who have not been convicted of a crime is a national trend. According to the Pretrial Justice Institute (2013), on a typical day in the United States six out of ten jail inmates are awaiting trial, *not* serving a sentence for a conviction. Flying in the face of the core American values of "innocent until proven guilty" and "justice and equality for all," higher-income individuals who have committed serious crimes are likely to be freed on bail while low-income individuals who have committed less serious crimes remain incarcerated because they are unable to pay. Once they come to trial, individuals who are already incarcerated before their trial are more likely to be sentenced to prison than individuals who were out on bail, regardless of the crime.

———

There is some encouraging evidence from across the United States that rates of incarceration are declining. California, the state with the largest number of people behind bars, was ordered by a panel of federal judges to reduce the state's prison population by approximately 10,000 to deal with prison over-crowding. Nationally, incarceration rates are going down for black men and women and for white men (but not for white women). Declining incarceration rates can be attributed to various factors, including changing social attitudes regarding drugs (particularly marijuana); large numbers of inmates finishing the lengthy mandatory sentences they were ordered to serve at the height of the War on Drugs in the 1980s and 1990s; budgetary constraints, including the rising cost of prison health care as prisoners age; and the ongoing advocacy work of community and prisoners' rights organizations.

However, the long-term impact of thirty years of mass incarceration will continue to resonate for millions of Americans (Comfort 2007; Leverentz 2014). After paying their dues to society, formerly incarcerated individuals continue to experience loss of parental rights; exclusion from public housing for themselves and family members; loss of access to government benefits such as TANF; discriminatory hiring practices; impaired access to assistance for higher education; deportation; disqualification from serving in the military, holding government jobs, or obtaining a variety of permits and licenses; and loss of eligibility to vote—this last a particularly egregious instance of loss of power and autonomy (cf. Uggen, Shannon, & Manza 2012). Nationwide, 40 percent of prisoners reenter prison within three years of release (Pew Center on the States 2011). More immediately relevant for Isabella, 52.8 percent of the 816 women released in 1995 from the main Massachusetts prison for women (MCI-Framingham) were back in prison at least once by the year 2010.[6]

A large-scale study of former prisoners found that 80 percent of men and 90 percent of women had chronic health problems that required treatment or management; 39 percent of men and 62 percent of women reported multiple health problems; 14 percent of men and 22 percent of women had physical health problems severe enough to qualify for and receive disability pensions (Mallik-Kane & Visher 2008). Even when controlling for wages, race, and other key demographic factors, incarceration's harmful impact on health not only remains powerful but exceeds the impact of other factors commonly used to explain health disparities, including health insurance status (Massoglia 2008b; Schnittker & John 2007). A retrospective study of all inmates released from the Washington State Department of Corrections between 1999 and 2003 uncovered a risk of death among former inmates that was 3.5 times that of other state residents. Especially notable, during the first two weeks after release the risk of death was 12.7 *times* higher than that of other state residents (Binswanger et al.). Recently published analysis of data from the National Longitudinal Survey of Youth indicates that the relationship between incarceration and mortality is significantly stronger for women than for men. The odds of dying post-release are *five times higher among women than among men.* "Even in the presence of many control variables significantly related to mortality [including race, parental education level, marital status, poverty status, employment status, and drug use], a robust relationship remains between incarceration and premature mortality for women, but not for men" (Massoglia 2014).

American men remain incarcerated at twenty times the rate of women. And as Isabella and Gloria know well, the legacy of their imprisonment continues to play out in the lives of their families and communities long after prison garb has been traded in for street clothes. Prison culture amplifies the sexist attitudes and gender violence of so-called free society. Three decades of mass incarceration in which large numbers of men have been locked up in violent and hypermasculine institutions has wreaked havoc on entire communities, putting women at great risk of becoming the victims of the rage and frustration of men immersed in prison culture.

Structural barriers created by misguided policies add fuel to the fire. Many men exit prison to find themselves barred from ever obtaining employment in the legal economy, unable to afford stable housing, and unable to support their families. When men leave jail, they compete with women for the limited number of (typically low-paying) jobs available in low-income communities that already experience high unemployment rates. Barriers to employment for former prisoners are driven by social stigma and lack of work experience, and by laws permitting or even mandating criminal background checks, a practice that puts men (who are more likely than women to have a criminal record) at a disadvantage. Setting the stage for gendered animosity, welfare eligibility tends to be limited to poor women with children; and nearly all Section VIII subsidized housing vouchers (housing subsidies for low-income households) go to female-headed households. Because state and federal laws exclude individuals holding criminal records from eligibility for public and subsidized housing, people released from prison (who are, again, more likely to be men than women, given the demographics of incarceration) often find that they are dependent on women for a roof over their heads. However, the same law allows (and sometimes requires) law-abiding citizens to be evicted if a former prisoner or someone who commits a crime is caught staying in their house. Several of the Boston women lost their housing because a man—even if he was their children's father—moved into their apartment, with or without their consent. Yet a low-income man who has to pay his own rent is unlikely to be able to pay child support, which legitimately enrages the mothers. Failure to pay child support, in turn, can be used by the courts as a reason to send a parent to jail, which legitimately enrages (for the most part) fathers. In short, policies and laws that pit women and men against each other are a setup for keeping too many Americans locked into the prison system.

Reflecting our broad American focus on individual flaws rather than on the structural conditions that lead to misery, the promotion of competition, conflict, and polarization along gender lines shifts attention away from broad social and economic inequalities to the wrongs committed by individual members of the so-called "opposite sex." From this perspective, institutional policies and cultures obscure underlying power regimes, militate against the formation of group or class-consciousness and inhibit the development of collective action.

A few months before this writing, Isabella called to tell us that four people she knew had died of overdoses in the previous week. All had just been released from prison. We asked if she could help us understand why the War on Drugs has not worked. "Locking people up doesn't help. People get out and have nowhere to go. Their family is fed up and don't understand. . . . They just don't get it. They say [drug use] is a choice. But locking them up just shows them how to be better criminals." Her voice trailing off, Isabella added, "or dead."

Conclusion

The Real Questions and a Blueprint for Moving Forward

> To find theories of theodicy or salvational hopes in the very same institutions which
> were responsible for creating the conditions for these sufferings in the first place, is an
> exercise of subtle power that locks the victims of violence and injustice into frozen
> positions.
>
> —Veena Das, "Suffering, Theodicies, Disciplinary Practices, Appropria-
> tions" (2010)

These are the questions that annoy and confound judges, social workers, doctors, correctional officers, and policy makers: Why are women like Francesca
and Kahtia so stuck in their misery despite the enormous amount of resources
our society puts into assisting, treating, and punishing them? There are programs out there to help them: job-training programs, battered women's
programs, mental health programs, housing programs, parenting programs,
welfare programs, and substance abuse programs. All of the women who
participated in this project rely on doctors for medication; all have seen multiple therapists and caseworkers; all have attended numerous Twelve Step
meetings; all have received treatment in rehabilitation programs both within-
and out of prison; almost all have called on the police and the courts to restrain
a violent boyfriend or family member; and all have received some sort of
financial assistance from the government.

Why do the women choose not to finish the programs, follow through with
what they learned, or change their attitudes? In the words of more than one
caseworker: Why do they "take one step forward and two steps back?" They
have had Twelve Step sponsors and instruction; they can choose to own up to
their addiction and commit to abstinence. And they have had enough contact

with the correctional system to know that if they "self-medicate," they will end up in jail. So why do they persist in choosing to use illicit drugs? Yes, they were victims of trauma, but they have been treated for PTSD. Why don't they choose to move on? Other people do. They all have had therapy. They know that women need to learn to develop more autonomy. No one forces them to enter one lousy, violent relationship after another. In the year 2013 we have rape crisis hotlines and the Violence Against Women Act. Surely the women know that if they choose to sleep on the street or trade sex for money or drugs, they are bound to be assaulted.

Why do they make such bad choices?

The questions we ask say a great deal about how the asker sees the world, and the ways in which we ask these questions dictate the possible answers. When we ask why some women persist in making bad choices, we assume that their past choices led to their current situation—that the miseries they experience are a consequence of their personal (bad) choices rather than of luck or of structural forces. We assume the availability of real choices—not only the ersatz choice to change one's attitude. We assume that all individuals actually have the freedom to make choices, an assumption that most certainly is not valid for prisoners and not necessarily valid for Americans who live in poverty, with disabilities, or with race or gender discrimination. We assume that "good" individual choices will have good outcomes—an assumption far from self-evident in this era of reduced social and economic mobility. The doctrine of choice dictates that battered women can and should leave their batterers (notwithstanding the real possibility that they have no place to go); that women should make better choices in their boyfriends (notwithstanding, as Elizabeth has commented, that employed, reliable, upstanding men are not interested in women like her); that they should choose good jobs rather than sex work or shoplifting (notwithstanding that the triple whammy of poor education, a criminal record, and economic recession make it unlikely that they will earn a living wage); that they should stay out of unsafe neighborhoods (notwithstanding pervasive racial segregation and policies that concentrate low-income housing in economically blighted neighborhoods); that they should not take illicit drugs (notwithstanding the broad American consensus that drugs are the best way to deal with pain). And the doctrine of choice disregards the vicissitudes of chance that affect all of us and to which those who are ill or weak or powerless are especially vulnerable.

Over the past five years we have learned that the choice to leave the home of a sexually abusive stepfather thrusts many young women onto the streets and into the juvenile detention circuit in which sexual violence is rampant. The choice to leave an abusive boyfriend or husband does not preclude a subsequent abusive relationship in a community in which large numbers of men have spent time in the hypermasculine incubators of jails and prisons. The choice to call the police can backfire when the woman herself is locked up because of an outstanding warrant. The choice to join a job-training program will not put a woman on the track to economic independence if potential employers tag her, in Tonya's words, as "an angry black woman with a do-rag" and come up with an array of reasons not to hire her. Even landing a job does not guarantee progress if the only jobs available pay minimum wage with no hope of advancement, and if women are fired for taking time off to care for sick children or elderly parents. We have learned that the choice to own up to one's own faults does not alter the structural inequalities that limit one's options to "crap, crappier, and crappiest. So what are you going to choose?" (Dunn and Powell-Williams 2007, p. 999). And we have learned that when women resist the practices of one powerful institution, they are likely to find themselves smack in the arms of another, equally powerful one.

Throughout this book we argue that medicalization and criminalization are complementary devices for operationalizing and enforcing the grand narrative of personal choice. The United States excels at both devices. We boast both the highest incarceration rate in the world and the highest usage of prescription medication. And while medicine sounds more benign than prison, both focus on changing the individual rather than changing the social conditions that cause distress. Mad or bad, treat or punish: these often are false dichotomies that propel women like Elizabeth and Gloria ever deeper into an institutional circuit in which the dominant ethos is the same as in the outside world—gender polarization, racism, the belief that poverty is inevitable and that suffering is a consequence of personal flaws.

It is a short hop from portraying suffering as the consequence of an individual's flaws to the criminalization of suffering and the incarceration of sufferers. Poor and homeless women are told that their problems are caused by mental illness, addiction, procrastination, and the inability to follow through on bureaucratic paperwork. They are encouraged to develop self-esteem, stand up for themselves, comply with doctors' orders, follow through on regimes of antidepressants and antipsychotics, admit their powerlessness, take responsibility for their failures, and turn themselves over to a Higher Power. Even in Massachusetts—albeit at a far slower pace than in most other states—when women such as Isabella and Joy "fail" to respond to "treatment," they are sent to prison for discipline, punishment, and reform, further propelling the cycle of unemployability, homelessness, and misery. It is no coincidence that the country with the highest per capita rate of prescription and over-the-counter medication usage and the highest per capita spending on health care also has the highest rate of incarceration in the world.

The perceived dichotomy of "treating" versus "punishing" reflects an inability or unwillingness to look beyond the cult of individualism for the causes and solutions to suffering. The fervor with which poverty and victimization are treated as an individual status obscures the structural inequalities that give rise to those very conditions. Most of the Boston women say that they do not have friends; they have only associates. When we ask what the difference is, we are told, "A friend is someone I can trust." Associates, in contrast, are people with whom one gets high or the people with whom one has been involuntarily connected in prison or other institutions. On the ground, in myriad explicit and implicit ways, social policies and cultural attitudes push women into being afraid of and not trusting men; push men into being resentful of women's greater access to welfare and housing; and push blacks and whites toward blaming each other for their problems. Even within homogenous race and gender categories there are institutional pressures to spy on and distrust one's fellow sufferers in prisons and therapeutic communities where Joy and others in her situation are rewarded for reporting infractions committed by others. In the end, each person is led to believe that one's misery is one's alone, a stance that militates against the formation of group, race, or class consciousness, and inhibits the desire and ability to work collectively to change the system.

THE REAL QUESTIONS

Perhaps we have posed the wrong questions. Rather than asking why these particular individuals continue to suffer despite all of the treatment and correction they receive, perhaps we need to ask why we prefer investing in curing diseases over supporting healthy communities. Why as a society are we willing to live with the social inequalities, poverty, environmental pollution, and violence against women and children that generate misery? Why are we willing to lock up millions of men and women for the crime of having been damaged by social failings? Why do we allow so many among us to remain mired in suffering, in the caste of the ill and afflicted?

On an empirical level, there are many who profit financially from the misery of Americans like the women described in this book. Drug cartels, pharmaceutical companies, lawyers, and the massive correctional, service, and therapeutic industries make their living—from the distress of others. The largest income for transnational organized crime comes from illicit drugs (UNODC 2011). According to Mexico's public safety secretary, drug cartels currently take in $64.34 billion from their sales to users in the United States (*Latin American Herald Tribune* 2013). The global pharmaceuticals market is worth $300 billion a year; the ten largest drugs companies control more than one-third of this market, with several amassing sales of more than $10 billion a year and profit margins as high as 30 percent (WHO 2013). The rapidly expanding privatization of prisons has also led to big profits. The Corrections Corporation of America recorded $1.7 billion in total revenue in 2011; Geo Group Inc. recorded $1.6 billion in the same year (Lee 2012). As Jill McCorkel (2013, p. 12) argues, "It is hardly coincidence that [private prison corporations are] promoting an ideology of addiction which holds that drug-involved offenders can never be 'cured,'" but rather will need treatment and correction for the rest of their lives. Internationally and nationally there are powerful interest groups intent on maintaining the lucrative status quo.

On a deeper level, we Americans desperately want to believe that all people have a chance and, if things don't work out, then the anomaly has to be the person who didn't do enough or try enough or somehow just wasn't good enough or strong enough. If, as is the case in the United States today, misery is understood to be the result of personal flaws (genetic flaws, in particular, have become a popular explanation for a wide range of miseries) or bad choices (including the choice not to recover from trauma), then the rest of us don't need to try to change the system. We just need to, as the self-help movement says, "work on ourselves." And if suffering is a personal matter, then the social obligation to provide succor to others is even smaller, easily replaced by punishing those who made the bad choices in the first place. This policy direction both fits the conservative "fiscal responsibility and small government" mantra and serves the didactic value of showing what happens to those who make the "wrong" choices. As Jeremy Seabrook (2002, p. 97) argues, "The underclass has a useful function in a society where most conceive of themselves as middle class. They serve as a warning to keep the rest of us in line. . . . They impose a salutary discipline on the majority, a powerful encouragement to keep us to beaten pathways, lest our fate come to resemble theirs."

The women we have come to know over the past five years are "neither angels nor demons" (Ferraro 2006). Like all of us, they are sometimes mean-spirited or selfish, and they make their share of mistakes. And, like all of us, they deeply love their children, they feel good when they can help others, and they try to look forward to a happier future. The reason that Francesca, Kahtia, Anasia, and Isabella can't catch a break is *not* because they are, in some essential way, different from "us." To the contrary, they are, canaries in the coal mine in an era when our tunnel-vision focus on medication and criminalization as solutions to human misery obscures the harshness of economic ideologies that allow the rich to become richer and the poor to become poorer, deflects attention from social ideologies that promote gender and racial conflict, and absolves government and corporate leadership from instituting policies and enforcing regulations that reduce poverty, racism, and sexual violence.

MOVING FORWARD: FROM THE PROBLEM OF THE NEEDY TO THE RIGHTS AT ALL HUMAN BEINGS

Five years of following a group of women through one of the best-funded, well-intentioned, and well-informed institutional circuits in the United States have made clear to us that our national commitment to ensuring that all members of society have access to housing, education, good nutrition, and bodily safety is neither consistent nor vigorous. That lack of commitment translates into programs that come and go at the whims of politicians, charitable organizations, and budget offices. It translates into the absurdity that SSI and TANF do not provide sufficient funds for basic necessities, essentially forcing Americans deemed eligible for these programs to break the rules or even break the law in order to cover the expenses of daily life. It translates into the absence of sustained efforts to enable all Americans to have homes, and it translates into homeless shelter rules that keep individuals moving from one facility to the next. It translates into battered women's shelters that provide short-term sanctuary from a violent partner but do not provide the financial resources to make it possible for a woman to set up a life for herself and her children independent of male support. And it results in the majority of frontline workers in the institutional circuit being underpaid, overworked, and asked to do the impossible: to "cure" the suffering caused by violence and inequality.

Reliance solely on interventions aimed at correcting the individual cannot prevent the growth of the caste of the ill and afflicted. Without sustained efforts to eliminate poverty, racism, and sexual violence, the United States will continue to produce new caste members. Recognizing the deep and complex connections between social inequality and suffering, we note that there are programs and policies that can serve as national models for moving forward.

We urge communities as well as state and federal governments to adopt models of restorative justice in place of the current victim-versus-perpetrator model on which the penal system rests. Using techniques such as mediation and circles of support, restorative justice acknowledges that both the victim and the surrounding community have been affected by the action of the offender, emphasizes the offender's obligation to make amends and repair the damage caused by the offense, provides victims a direct say in the judgment process, and addresses steps that the community can take to reduce further offense and injustice (Zehr & Mika 1998; for an excellent assessment of restorative justice as a tool in addressing violence against women, see Ptacek 2010).

We also commend programs such as Cambridge Health Alliance's Victims of Violence that not only provide therapy but also recognize and address the ongoing dangers faced by clients, as well as the need for community-based action to prevent violence and repair the suffering caused by violence (see Herman 1997). As Francesca announced the first time we met her, we need to tell our politicians to "stop standing by" while people live on the street. While it is not without problems, we believe that the "housing first" model in which vulnerable individuals and families are quickly placed into permanent housing is a step in the right direction. It simply is not feasible for individuals and families to pull other aspects of their lives together in the absence of safe and secure housing.

More broadly, we believe that by shifting the public conversation from the "problems of the needy" to the "rights of all human beings," we can encourage the development of long-term, cohesive, adequately funded public institutions. What we are calling for is a change from the Medicaid model of providing assistance to individuals who can prove to the satisfaction of the state that they are truly needy, to the Medicare model of acknowledging that all human beings are vulnerable to illness and old age and deserve the support of their fellow human beings.

While the United States remains stuck in debates over how to tweak or refine our individualized approach to suffering (e.g., Shall we send drug users to jail, drug court, or psychiatric treatment hospitals? Shall we expand Medicaid to those earning less than 138 percent of the federal poverty line of $11,484, or limit it to those earning under the federal poverty line?), the international community has developed powerful frameworks that spell out the responsibility of the state to respect, protect, and fulfill human rights. Adopted by the United Nations General Assembly on December 10, 1948, the Universal Declaration of Human Rights defines the rights and freedoms to which all people are inalienably entitled regardless of sex, national or ethnic origin, race, religion, language, or other status. By virtue of being human, each of us is born with and possesses the right to basic minimum standards of food, housing, health care, and safety; the right to make free and informed choices in all spheres of life—including sexuality, reproduction, marriage, family formation, and the timing and spacing of children; the right to have access to the information, means, and security needed to exercise voluntary choice; and the right to liberty and freedom of expression.[1]

Human rights are realized through specific policies and concrete institutions, through economic principles and legislative measures that reduce inequality, and through the development of agencies and programs that truly attend to the suffering caused by inequalities rather than simply putting Band-Aids on the wounds. The experiences of the Boston women have made clear the need for integrated efforts that address both the causes and the consequences of suffering as embedded in a single social system. International human rights conventions proclaim that human rights—whether relating to civil, cultural, economic, political, or social issues—are indivisible, interdependent, and interrelated. When an individual's rights are violated in one sphere, there invariably is spillover into other spheres. Thus, we see that the violation of Elizabeth's right to housing led to the violation of her right to bodily safety; the violation of Francesca's and of Joy's right to their own bodily integrity led to the violation of their right to health; for Isabella the violation of her liberty led to the violation of her right to raise her children; for Anasia, the violation of her right to an education led to the violation of her right to fulfill the basic minimum standards of housing.

Human rights can be addressed and vouchsafed only through identifying the causes of poverty, injustice, and misery; empowering rights-holders (all human beings) to claim their rights; and requiring duty-bearers (governments, powerful organizations and institutions, and all those in possession of might and resources) to meet their obligations. We believe it is crucial for the United States to ratify and *enforce* the treaties that spell out the rights of all human beings. Two documents of particular relevance to the Boston women are the United Nations Convention on the Elimination of All Forms of Discrimination Against Women and the United Nations Rules for the Treatment of Women Prisoners and Non-custodial Measures for Women Offenders.

Laws and treaties may seem far removed from the day-to-day suffering of the women we have described in this book. After all, the Violence Against Women Act was not only passed—it was also renewed—and it hasn't stopped Joey from spitting on Francesca, John from locking Gloria in her room, or a procession of thugs from beating on Ginger. This dilemma is not new, but neither is it reasonable to throw up our hands in defeat. In 1963, the Reverend Dr. Martin Luther King Jr. said:

> Now the . . . myth that gets around is the idea that legislation cannot really solve the problem and that it has no great role to play in this period of social change because you've got to change the heart and you can't change the heart through legislation. You can't legislate morals. The job must be done through education and religion. Well, there's a half-truth involved here. Certainly, if the problem is to be solved then in the final sense, hearts must be changed. Religion and education must play a great role in changing the heart. But we must go on to say that while it may be true that morality cannot be legislated, behavior can be regulated. It may be true that the law cannot change the heart but it can restrain the heartless. It may be true that the law cannot make a man love me but it can keep him from lynching me and I think that is pretty important, also."

APPENDIX

Methodology and Project Participant Overview

From March through August 2008 we spent time at two Boston facilities that provide services to poor, homeless, or recently incarcerated women. During those months we shared our interest in enlisting women in a five-year project in which they would receive a monthly incentive (a monthly pass on the mass-transit system or a $20 CVS gift card) in return for staying in touch with us and allowing us to speak with them about what was happening in their lives. Women were told that they could withdraw from the project at any time or refuse to answer any question without penalty or further interrogation and that they would continue to receive the incentive. Forty-seven women joined the project. At the end of four years twenty-six remained regularly involved in the project; twenty-three women continued to be actively involved for all five years; about half that number remain in touch with us today.

Throughout this book names and identifying details have been changed to protect anonymity. This project received ethics approval from the Suffolk University Institutional Review Board and from the directors of the facilities where we recruited participants.

Between 2008 and 2013, we strove to meet with each project participant once a month for an informal chat and once every three months for a more structured conversation. We accompanied some of the women to court hearings and other appointments, and we visited some of them at their homes. We also saw the women at the various places they frequented, such as parks, programs, churches, and shelters.

This project involved both ethnographic work and semistructured interviews. The first week of each month we touched base with the women to give them their incentives and remind them that we are still interested in them. Every three months we conducted semistructured in-depth interviews covering recent employment, education, family, relationships, children, health, drug use, criminal activity, and life events (including short- and long-term goals). The ethnographic component involved informal contact with the women at locations and events of their choosing. As the study progressed, some women invited us to christenings, birthdays, weddings, court hearings, graduations, and family events and to visit them in the hospital. At these events our goal was to support the women and gain a broader, contextualized understanding of their experiences. Over time we have come to know many of their family members and close friends. While we welcomed the comments and conversations of these other people, our focus always remained the project participants.

Because the establishment of close relationships was central to this project, each woman maintained contact only with Susan or Maureen, depending on which of us she had met first. To streamline the book's narrative, we use the first-person plural pronoun throughout (for example, "Each time we met Elizabeth . . ."), though only one of us actually met with any particular woman.

Staying in touch with project participants for five years proved a logistical challenge, and we came to understand why there are so few long-term studies of similar populations. No woman remained at the same address or retained the same phone number over the five years of the study. Some of the women had as many as twenty different phone numbers, and for part or all of the project period many had no address where they could be reached. Many used more than one name (especially when dealing with the institutional circuit), and most of the women disappeared for at least a while during periods of heavy drug use ("drug runs"). We attribute the success we have had in keeping in touch to several factors. First is the monthly incentive; a mass-transit pass made it possible for the women to get to their numerous appointments and to experience some degree of freedom in moving around the Boston area. Second, we have made conscious efforts not to judge the women or their actions. For example, we reiterated that "we don't care if you are using drugs or not. We just want you to be happy and safe." While we may not have convinced all of the women that we are not social workers, we believe that most of the women (like most people everywhere) appreciated our genuine interest and concern. Third, we have made ourselves accessible to the women at some of the facilities they frequent and in our offices. Suffolk University is located in downtown Boston quite near a large park (the Boston Common) and a variety of service and welfare agencies that the women use. Especially when homeless, many of the women came to appreciate the clean restrooms in our office building. And fourth, we met the women in locations of their choosing, including a coffee shop or restaurant where we could sit and relax over a shared meal. While all of us enjoy a nice lunch, a restaurant meal is a particular treat for women who rely on food stamps and homeless shelters for food.

Throughout the project, it was a challenge to work with women who have had extensive contact, often for years or even decades, with caseworkers, therapists, and other representatives of the institutional circuit who have drilled them in the right things to say in order to get welfare benefits, get out of jail, or simply to make a good impression. We are well aware that the unequal power dynamics of our relationships infuse all of our interactions. We are educated, white, and middle-class; we own cars, are securely housed, are relatively healthy; we're the ones asking rather than answering questions, and we're the distributors of monthly incentives.

Both the most difficult and the most rewarding aspects of a long-term project of this sort are the personal relationships we have developed with the women. As researchers it has been frustrating to work with individuals who have trouble remembering to come to meetings, who sometimes are too doped up on prescription or street drugs to make much sense, who may still think that we will reward them if they tell us that they are doing the "right things," and who have learned in the institutional circuit that it is often best not to reveal the truth about various aspects of their lives. More important, it pained us deeply when the women told us about horrible things that happened to them, when we saw their bruises during visits to the hospital after a rape or assault, when their children were taken away from them, and when we heard from friends or family members that they had been locked up. We feel some satisfaction knowing that our office became a safe space for women who have few places in which they can feel secure, and we know that for a few of the women our presence in their lives has been a source of stability or even pride.

As the project came toward its end, we explained to the participants that while we would no longer do formal interviews or give out mass-transit passes, our doors will always be open to them, and they can call us on our office or cell phones. It is our intention to follow the lead of each individual woman regarding how deeply involved she wishes to remain with us. While we expect that most will slowly drift away once we no longer frequent the institutional circuit or give out monthly incentives, we know that we have developed some ties that transcend the researcher-subject relationship and that have become true friendships. Francesca knows that she can count on us to continue to come and give her a ride when her boyfriend kicks her out of his house; Joy knows we will continue to cry with her when she is raped or beaten; and Kahtia knows that we will keep coming around her house for her rice and beans and for the hugs her daughters give to Auntie Susan and Auntie Maureen.

In line with current practice, we have explained our findings and recommendations to the women individually and in small groups, and we have asked for their feedback throughout the process of writing this book. We take seriously our obligation to advocate for the women and their community, and we welcome opportunities to speak on their behalf in academic, policy, and community venues.

PROJECT PARTICIPANTS

All of the initial forty-seven study participants had been incarcerated for at least one night in the year preceding the start of the project. *Of the twenty-six women who remained in the project for at least four years, twelve were reincarcerated during that time.*

The basic demographic characteristics of the study participants are similar to those of all women incarcerated in Massachusetts as of January 1, 2008 (table 2). The median age of the initial forty-seven study participants in 2008 was 38 (versus 37 years old for

TABLE 2   COMPARATIVE DEMOGRAPHIC CHARACTERISTICS
OF PROJECT VOLUNTEERS VERSUS WOMEN INCARCERATED IN
MASSACHUSETTS AS OF JANUARY 1, 2008

	Women in Project ($n = 47$)	All incarcerated females in Massachusetts ($n = 607$)
Median age (years)	38	37
Marital status (percentage)		
Single	57.4	58.8
Ever Married	42.6	41.2
Race (percentage)		
White	71.7	63.9
Black	19.6	16.1
Other	8.7	19.2
Education (percentage)		
Less than high school	42.6	40.5
Completed high school, plus	57.4	59.5
Criminal offense (percentage)		
Person	13.0	34.4
Property	17.4	17.8
Drugs	37.0	31.1
Other	10.9	15.1

SOURCE FOR MASSACHUSETTS STATISTICS: Massachusetts Department of Corrections 2008.

women incarcerated in Massachusetts overall; McLaughlin 2008). At the time we began the study, 34 percent of the women were age 41 or older; 43 percent were age 31–40; 23 percent were age 20–30. The majority (72%) of the study women were white, 20 percent were black, and 8 percent were Hispanic or Asian. White women were slightly overrepresented in our project, as were older women. In Massachusetts 64 percent of women inmates in 2008 were white. Because of Boston-area demographics and the settings where we initially met the project participants (public facilities), as well as cultural and language barriers that likely discouraged non-English-speaking women from joining the project, very few Hispanic women participated. We suggest that readers look to work by Juanita Diaz-Cotto in order to gain a fuller understanding of the experiences of Latinas with the correctional system.

Thirty-eight percent of project participants were raised by both biological parents. Forty-three percent were raised by their mother, and 13 percent by grandparents. Eleven had been in foster care as children or in a juvenile residential institution. Twenty-one had left home by age sixteen, most commonly because of abuse.

Fifty-seven percent of the study women did not finish high school. While we did not measure literacy, several of the women seemed to struggle with reading forms and announcements. Overall, 33 percent of women incarcerated in Massachusetts enter the Department of Corrections with less than a ninth-grade reading level, and 38 percent with less than a sixth-grade math level. Male inmates are in even poorer shape: 45 percent enter the DOC with less than a ninth-grade reading level, and 44 percent with less than a sixth-grade math level (Research and Planning Division 2013, p. 17).

Forty-three percent of the women have been married at some point in their lives, though only five women were married at the time this study began. All had been, and currently were, involved with boyfriends (in several cases, girlfriends), fiancés, or fathers of their children. All but two of the women have children. The median number of live births at the time the project started was two, and the median age that a woman first gave birth was nineteen.

At the time the project began, less than one-third of the women had worked steadily at legal jobs throughout most of their adult lives. *Of the twenty-six women who remained in the project for at least four years, only four were steadily employed for most of that period. Twenty-two received SSI, SSDI, or TANF (welfare) payments.*

Thirty-two women had experienced extended periods of homelessness in the years prior to the start of the study. *Of the twenty-six women who remained in the project for at least four years, only nine were securely housed for most of that period.*

In our initial interviews, forty-one of the women reported drug addiction (87%), and twenty-seven (57%) defined themselves as alcoholics. All reported some level of mental health struggle and 85 percent had received formal mental illness diagnoses before the project began. Depression, anxiety disorder, PTSD, and bipolar disorder were the four most frequently reported mental illnesses. *Of the twenty-six women who remained in the project for at least four years, twenty-two reported receiving prescriptions for some sort of psychiatric medication during that period.*

At the time the project started, 81 percent of the women reported a chronic physical illness (hepatitis C, asthma, back pain, arthritis, unresolved gynecological problems, high blood pressure, heart disease, liver disease, hepatitis B, HIV, chronic headaches, severe tooth decay). *Of the twenty-six women who remained in the project for at least four years, twenty were hospitalized overnight at least once during that period.*

The size of the study population is not large enough for us to generalize about differences in life experiences associated with race or any other demographic characteristic. We do note that the black women who joined this project were somewhat more likely than the white women to stay in touch with us throughout the full five years, more likely to maintain family ties, and more likely to struggle with literacy. We also note that the older women were somewhat more likely than the younger women to make obtaining permanent housing a top priority.

The number of participants does not allow us to reach significant conclusions regarding differences between the women who stayed in the project for most or all of the five years and women who dropped out or disappeared after one or two meetings. We do note a few interesting trends. Women whose most recent incarceration was for a drug or alcohol offense were far more likely to stay in the project than women whose most recent incarceration was a crime against a person or a property offense. Black women, less educated women, and older women were more likely than white women, more educated women, or younger women to stick with the project. The median age of the women who stayed was 40; the median age of those who did not was 29. There were no other obvious demographic differences between the two groups.

NOTES

1. This is true even when age, race, education, and marital and employment status are taken into account (Massoglia 2008b).

2. For more than a century, scholars have debated whether the designation *caste* makes sense only in terms of traditional Indian society, or whether the term can be used more broadly to describe highly stratified societies found in a number of places around the world. We have chosen not to enter into that debate here. Indian scholar Ursula Sharma (1999) cogently argues that we turn our attention to process rather than structure, and think about "castification" as a social and political process by which ethnic or other groups become part of a rank ordering of some kind. "If we think in terms of process rather than form we do not have to get bogged down in the problem of whether a group is a 'caste' or a 'tribe' but can focus on the more constructive question of the direction in which current change is moving" (p. 93).

3. The Government Accountability Office estimates that at least 2.4 million young adults aged eighteen through twenty-six—or 6.5 percent of the noninstitutionalized young adults in that age range—had a serious mental illness in 2006, and they had lower levels of education on average than other young adults. The actual number is likely to be higher than 2.4 million because homeless, institutionalized, and incarcerated persons (groups with potentially high rates of mental illness) were not included in this estimate.

CHAPTER 1

1. Hepatitis C is a complicated illness. Chronic infection is often asymptomatic, though 70 percent of those infected develop chronic liver disease over the following twenty to thirty years. The most common symptoms include nausea, fatigue, and

abdominal pain. Diagnosis is also complicated, with multiple tests often necessary over an extended period of time to confirm that a person has the disease and whether it is active. This presents challenges particularly to incarcerated women, who generally serve shorter prison terms than men. The common treatment is a combination of Interferon and other drugs. Serious side-effects of this drug regimen include headaches, loss of appetite, hair loss, muscle and joint pain, and suppression of immune defense, which may result in susceptibility to other infections. Other side-effects include insomnia, anxiety, and depression. Sustained positive response to treatment (cure or long-term remission) occurs in only 15 to 20 percent of patients (G. Davis 2002).

2. Beth Richie (2012) tracks the transition away from 1960s grassroots feminist organizations that opened shelters and rape crisis centers as an integral part of a wider program of political activism aimed at battling gender oppression. In the wake of the conservative ethos that became dominant in the country during the 1970s and 1980s, the movement to combat violence against women increasingly pursued "a safer, less antagonistic strategy," and its advocates developed a professional identity as "specialists" who work with battered women (Richie 2012, p. 75). As battered women's shelters became part of the mainstream institutional circuit, emphasis shifted from working together for social change to teaching women that they should take responsibility for improving their own situations and requiring women to apply for government services (Bumiller 2008).

3. In 2009 Wayne County, Michigan, prosecutor Kym Worthy discovered more than 11,303 rape kits that had been used by hospitals to collect DNA evidence sitting on shelves in a warehouse. The kits had never been tested. Not only could the DNA evidence have led to arrests that might have prevented further rapes, but the original victims had undergone the intrusive vaginal probing for nothing (Garcia, Powers, & Hopper 2013).

4. Despite rape shield laws designed to protect women from verbal assaults by defense lawyers at rape trials, victims can be asked about their social and sexual history when these issues are ruled relevant to determining consent.

CHAPTER 2

1. Neo-Synephrine is an over-the-counter nasal spray. We guess Elizabeth means norepinephrine, a neurotransmitter in the brain.

2. During the coldest winter months, Boston-area shelters relax policies that keep homeless people out of the shelter during the day.

3. This rate of emergency rooms use is substantially higher than that for the general population. A recent study of emergency room usage in 2009–2010 of patients who had made at least one visit to a primary care practice located in Boston Medical Center (the city hospital that the project women tend to frequent) found that most patients (65.4 percent) did not make any emergency room visits, 29.8 percent made occasional visits, and 4.9 percent made frequent (four or more) visits (Lasser 2012).

CHAPTER 3

1. Any race-based patterns that we identify among the women in this project must be understood in the broader context of overall higher rates of arrest and incarceration among African Americans vis-à-vis white Americans, despite research consistently showing that rates of drug abuse among whites are actually higher than among African Americans (L. T. Wu et al. 2011; Alexander 2012). Because the police as well as the courts seem slower to arrest and incarcerate white women, those white women who do end up in prison tend to be more troubled over longer periods of time than the black women.

2. Municipalities, counties, and states routinely ignore their legal obligations to affirmatively foster fair housing. As a consequence, even middle-class black families face barriers in moving away from poor and troubled neighborhoods (Lipsitz 2012).

3. In the first decade of the twenty-first century, for the first time in nearly forty years, there was a decline in the number of African Americans in prison—particularly African American women—and a steep rise in the number of white women going to prison. Among Hispanics the number of women imprisoned rose, and the number of men declined slightly (Mauer 2013).

4. This dynamic is, of course, exacerbated by broader social norms regarding racially segregated dating and family relationships. In particular, black women experience race-based exclusion from dating white men.

5. We are aware that women often told us what they thought we wanted to hear, and we believe that to be especially true in how black women spoke about race to us or in our presence. All of our interactions were shaped by the inequalities between the project women and us in power, status, class, and access to resources, and we are especially cognizant of the complexities of the racial dynamics and history of racism in the relationships between white researchers and black research subjects.

6. We thank George Lipsitz for this insight and wording.

CHAPTER 4

1. In a 2013 study, a team of scientists conducted a meta-analysis that examined methodologically solid studies of interventions for children diagnosed with PTSD. Out of 6,647 abstracts reviewed, the team found 21 trials and 1 cohort study that the scientists rated at low or medium risk of bias (in other words, these studies are sufficiently rigorous). The conclusion: no pharmacotherapy intervention demonstrated efficacy. Psychotherapy interventions showed slightly more promise, but "studies comparing interventions with active controls did not show benefit" (Forman-Hoffman et al. 2013, p. 534).

2. While she does not use the term, Ginger's memories of being hospitalized as a youth indicate that she was treated for gender identity disorder (GID), the formal psychiatric label used by psychologists and physicians to describe persons who experience

significant gender dysphoria (discontent with the biological sex they were born with). LGBTQ activists, as well as many psychologists, have advocated for eliminating GID from the *Diagnostic and Statistical Manual of Mental Disorders*, arguing that GID reinforces gender stereotypes by pathologizing behaviors and attitudes that violate the rigid gender dichotomy. Other feminist and queer writers have taken quite different positions on this issue (Stone 1991; Butler 1990). In the *DSM-V*, released in 2013, GID was replaced by the diagnosis "gender dysphoria." Both GID and gender dysphoria describe a condition in which someone is intensely uncomfortable with his or her biological gender and strongly identifies with, and wants to be, the opposite gender. In the *DSM-IV*, GID focused on the "identity" issue—namely, the incongruity between someone's birth gender and the gender with which he or she identifies. While this incongruity is still crucial to gender dysphoria, the drafters of the *DSM-V* wanted to emphasize the importance for diagnosis of *distress* about the incongruity. This shift reflects recognition that the disagreement between birth gender and identity may not necessarily be pathological if it does not cause the individual distress.

3. There is a strong consensus among researchers that individuals with various mental illnesses, including mood disorders, often self-medicate through illicit drugs (Swendsen et al. 2010). The women we know, as well as the social workers, correctional officers, and other professionals who work with them, frequently use the term "self-medication" in a negative sense. We wonder, What is the issue here? Is the problem the "self" part (in a society with a medical monopoly on drugs, one should not medicate oneself but rather be medicated by a doctor)? Or is the problem the "medicate" part (that is, some understanding that drugs do not change the underlying circumstances)? Interestingly, some of the women use the term "self-medicate" even in regard to legal drugs given by a doctor.

4. While psychoactive drugs certainly are necessary in many instances and frequently do increase autonomy rather than constrain it—for instance, a psychotic individual who is put on medication that allows her or him to actually function and think rationally—we emphasize that very few of the women in this study were diagnosed as psychotic. We also note that, due both to personal and institutional reasons, the women tended to stop and start medications quite abruptly. Sudden breaks in usage of psychiatric medication can be extremely harmful (Baldessarini et al. 2010).

5. Certain reforms have been made under President Barack Obama, most notably the Fair Sentencing Act of 2010 which reduces disparities in punishment for crack versus powder cocaine.

CHAPTER 5

1. Our blurring of doctors and therapists in this chapter is intentional. Typically, therapists refer the women to doctors for psychiatric medication, and doctors refer the women to therapists for talk therapy. The two disciplines, while based on rather different approaches, increasingly work in tandem, and the Boston women did not always know which provider was what. In the current era the links between talk therapy and

psychiatric medication have deepened both in popular culture and in professional practice. Although many psychotherapists reject what has become the dominant biological model of mental illness, the therapists, counselors, and caseworkers we interviewed in the course of this project were restricted to certain diagnostic categories set by the American Psychiatric Association so that insurance companies will cover a client's treatment or so that a client is ensured eligibility for Social Security or other social welfare programs. For the women of this project, psychiatry and psychotherapy (whether offered by a psychologist, a social worker, or some other type of mental health worker) are experienced as one system.

2. The women we work with have been "in the system" for decades. As a consequence, their ideas and explanations reflect what they have heard and been taught over many years in many different settings. Some of these ideas are no longer mainstream therapeutic beliefs and practices. Dana Becker (2005) notes that in her experience as a therapist, clients expected the therapeutic culture they learned on *Oprah* and from other pop culture sources.

3. We use the term "scientifically verifiable" in the standard sense of the scientific method as centering on experiments and outcomes that are consistently replicable regardless of who carries them out. In 2013, several weeks before the *DSM-V* was due to come out, the National Institute of Mental Health, the world's largest funding agency for mental health research, withdrew its support for the manual. NIMH director Thomas Insel (2013) criticized the *DSM*: "Unlike our definitions of ischemic heart disease, lymphoma, or AIDS, the *DSM* diagnoses are based on a consensus about clusters of clinical symptoms, not any objective laboratory measure." In place of categorizing symptoms, Insel argues, mental health research needs to focus on biological measures, genetics, and brain imaging that can be verified scientifically. While Insel's comments correctly identify a systematic weakness of the *DSM*, the alternative he suggests actually moves understandings of human suffering further away from actual experience and from social conditions, turning misery not only into a diagnostic category but into a scientifically measurable pathology.

4. While the public acceptance of physicians in the gatekeeping role is premised on the objectivity of science, there are significant differences among physicians and between eras in how they have ruled regarding Social Security Disability (Stone 1979). We also note that while we tend to assume that doctors' first and only loyalty is to their patients, in the current health care system, doctors generally are paid and employed by insurance companies, hospitals, and government agencies (including prisons).

5. Yehuda, Pratchett, and Pelcovitz (2012) argue that while PTSD may be a reasonable reaction to abuse or disaster, prolonged symptoms are likely to be linked to organic patterns in the individual's brain. Over the past decade the psychotherapeutic establishment increasingly has invoked genetic factors to explain the symptoms commonly related to PTSD. Since there are no current genetic treatments, this interpretative trend has not had an impact on the therapeutic management of the women with whom we have worked. We have noticed, however, that several of the women, including Elizabeth, speculate that their mental health problems are genetic.

CHAPTER 6

1. Weight is a complicated issue for the Boston women. While most buy into the general American belief that the ideal body is slim and that obesity is an "illness" and a visible sign of poor self-control and other character flaws, they depend on the carbo-hydrate-heavy meals at shelters and soup kitchens for sustenance, are (often) hooked on Pepsi for the sugar high to make it through the day, and are unable to pay for the gyms that sculpt the slim body shapes admired in American culture. Moreover, for drug users, being thin indicates that one is on a drug run (in fact, we have heard of parole officers cite weight loss as evidence of "relapse"); during periods of sobriety women try to gain their weight back in order to regain health.

2. In the long run Joy's dropping out probably did not impact her ability to pay back the loans. Ashley and Isabella, both of whom have far better educational and employ-ment histories than Joy, finished similar programs in medical assistance or medical billing, but could not find jobs due to their criminal records. Unfortunately, far too many educational institutions encourage students to take out loans for amounts that are a poor fit in terms of future earnings and become a lifelong burden to the former student.

3. We are intrigued with a relatively recent Twelve Step off-shoot called Underearn-ers Anonymous. While nowhere near as large an organization as AA, it does hold approximately ten daily meetings in California and New York and even England, Colom-bia, and Israel. UA's twelve "Symptoms of Underearning" all address the character flaws of the individual underearner; none refer to economic policies, recession, market forces, or the like. For the twelve symptoms, see www.underearnersanonymous.org.

4. We realize that our critique of Twelve Step programs will rub many readers the wrong way. To be clear, we have many friends and colleagues who believe that Twelve Step programs have helped them enormously. However, the women with whom we have conducted research have not found Twelve Step groups to be helpful in the long term. We suspect that Twelve Step programs may be more helpful for people who do have reasonable power over their own housing, safety, families, and freedom.

5. Some theologians and therapists have attempted to reinterpret the notion of powerlessness to mean mutuality, flexibility, or inherent strength (cf. Herndon 2001). We are not persuaded.

6. We are not in total agreement with Isabella's observation here. Two other proj-ect women, Vanessa and Ginger, told us on several occasions that "my mother is my higher power." Both of these women feel that their mother is "a wonderful person" who has "always been there for me."

7. Use of AA/NA in the correctional system is rarely challenged in terms of the First Amendment's Establishment Clause, which bars Congress from establishing a religion or making laws in regard to religion. It is challenged slightly more often on the basis of the Free Exercise Clause (also known as the Coercion Clause) (Sullivan 2009; Apanovitch 1998).

CHAPTER 7

1. Living with high levels of responsibility coupled with low levels of authority has been linked to poor health, chronic physical and mental distress, and greater risk of death (Marmot and Wilkinson 2006).

CHAPTER 8

1. The high rate of cesarean sections in the United States (over 30% of deliveries) is thought to be approximately twice that required by standard medical criteria, and is a classic example of medicalization, reflecting beliefs that women's bodies on their own are just not good enough, not competent enough, or not strong enough to give birth without medical intervention (Boston Women's Health Book Collective 2011; Childbirth Connection 2013; CDC 2011a).

2. Among the project participants, the black women were more likely to choose to serve out sentences rather than take on longer periods of intense supervision on parole or in pre-release facilities. Several black women told us that they might as well finish the sentence because parole officers would likely send them back to jail anyway (cf. Wood and May 2003).

3. According to a 2012 report by the Vera Institute of Justice (Henrichson & Delaney 2012), the total annual taxpayer cost of prisons in the forty states that provided data was $39 billion, and the average annual cost per inmate was $31,286. In Massachusetts, the average cost per year to house an inmate is $45,502.19 (Massachusetts Department of Corrections 2012).

4. The figures for male inmates were 24 percent classified as "open mental health cases" and 18 percent treated with psychiatric medication in prison (Massachusetts Department of Corrections 2013).

5. Further blurring the boundaries between medical and penal responses to suffering, Massachusetts General Laws, Chapter 123, Section 35, permits the courts to involuntarily commit to an inpatient substance abuse treatment program for a period of up to ninety days someone whose alcohol or drug use puts him- or herself or others at risk. In contrast to cases in which an individual is committed on the basis of psychiatric illness, Section 35 is carried out in criminal court with no possibility for appeal, and the final ruling is made by a judge, not a mental health expert (though a mental health expert offers an opinion). At least half a dozen of the women we have come to know have been "Section 35'd."

6. In contrast, in a study conducted by Glueck and Glueck early in the twentieth century of women charged with very similar crimes and released from the very same Massachusetts prison, only 16.3 percent were reincarcerated five years later (Glueck & Glueck 1934, cited in Norton-Hawk, Sered, & Mastrorilli 2013.)

CONCLUSION

1. The bulk of the writing about rights-based responses to suffering comes from the international community. The human rights language we use here is drawn primarily from the United Nations Population Fund.

REFERENCES

Aizer, Anna, and Doyle, Joseph J., Jr. 2011. "Juvenile Incarceration and Adult Outcomes: Evidence from Randomly-Assigned Judges." National Bureau of Economic Research Working Paper No. 19102. Issued June 2013. Retrieved from http://www.nber.org/papers/w19102.

Albrecht, James M. 2012. *Reconstructing Individualism: A Pragmatic Tradition from Emerson to Ellison.* New York: Fordham University Press.

Alexander, Michelle. 2012. *The New Jim Crow: Mass Incarceration in the Age of Colorblindness.* New York: The New Press.

American Bar Association and National Bar Association. 2001. Justice by Gender: The Lack of Appropriate Prevention, Diversion and Treatment Alternatives for Girls in the Justice System. Retrieved from http://www.americanbar.org/content/dam/aba/publishing/criminal_justice_section_newsletter/crimjust_juvjus_justicebygenderweb.authcheckdam.pdf.

Ames, Michael W., Lowe, Jennifer Dobruck, Dowd, Kelly, Liberman, Ruth J., and Youngblood, Deborah Connolly. 2013. *Massachusetts Economic Independence Index 2013.* Crittenton Women's Union. Retrieved from http://www.liveworkthrive.org/research_and_tools/reports_and_publications/Massachusetts_Economic_Independence_Index_2013.

Amnesty International. 1999. "Not Part of my Sentence: Violations of the Human Rights of Women in Custody." *United States of America, Rights for All.* Washington, D.C.

Anderson, G. 2004. *Chronic Conditions: Making the Case for Ongoing Care.* Baltimore: John Hopkins University Press.

Anderson, Gerard. 2010. "Chronic Care: Making the Case for Ongoing Care." Prepared for Robert Woods Johnson Foundation. Retrieved from http://www.rwjf.org/en/research-publications/find-rwjf-research/2010/01/chronic-care.html.

Angell, Marcia. 2011. "The Epidemic of Mental Illness: Why?" *New York Review of Books.* June 23. Retrieved from http://www.nybooks.com/articles/archives/2011/jun/23/epidemic-mental-illness-why/?page=1.

Apanovitch, Derek P. 1998. "Religion and Rehabilitation: The Requisition of God by the State." *Duke Law Journal* 47(4):785–852.

Appell, Annette R. 1998. "On Fixing 'Bad' Mothers and Saving Their Children." Pp. 356–380 in *"Bad" Mothers: The Politics of Blame in Twentieth-Century America.* Ed. Molly Ladd-Taylor and Lauri Umansky. New York: New York University Press.

Arriola, Kimberly J., Braithwaite, Ronald L., and Newkirk, Cassandra. 2006. *Health Issues among Incarcerated Women.* New Brunswick, NJ: Rutgers University Press.

Aston, Shaughney. 2009. "Identities Under Construction: Women Hailed as Addicts." *Health* (London) 13(6):611–628.

Auerhahn, Kathleen, and Leonard, Elizabeth Dermody. 2000. "Docile Bodies? Chemical Restraints and the Female Inmate." *Journal of Criminal Law and Criminology* 90(2):599–634.

Bader, Eleanor J. 2012a. Women Prisoners Endure Rampant Sexual Violence; Current Laws Not Sufficient. *Truthout.* December 21. Retrieved from http://truth-out.org/news/item/13280-women-prisoners-endure-rampant-s****l-violence-current-laws-not-sufficient.

Bader, Eleanor J. 2012b. "Women's Incarceration Rate Soars by over 600 Percent As They Face Abuse behind Bars. *Alternet.* December 23. Retrieved from http://www.alternet.org/civil-liberties/womens-incarceration-rate-soars-over-600-percent-they-face-abuse-behind-bars.

Baldessarini, Ross J., Tondo, Leonardo, Ghiani, Carmen, and Lepri, Beatrice. 2010. "Illness Risk following Rapid versus Gradual Discontinuation of Antidepressants." *American Journal of Psychiatry* 167(8):934–941.

Bancroft, R. Lundy, Silverman, Jay G., and Ritchie, Daniel. 2012. *The Batterer as Parent: Addressing the Impact of Domestic Violence on Family Dynamics.* 2nd ed. Los Angeles: Sage.

Bartky, Sandra Lee. 1990. *Femininity and Domination: Studies in the Phenomenology of Oppression.* New York: Routledge.

Batavia, Andrew I., and Beaulaurier, Richard L. 2001. "The Financial Vulnerability of People with Disabilities: Assessing Poverty Risks." *Journal of Sociology and Social Welfare* 28(1):139–162.

Becker, Dana. 2005. *The Myth of Empowerment: Women and the Therapeutic Culture in America.* New York: New York University Press.

Becker, Deborah, Mulvihill, Maggie and Stine, Rachel. 2012, December 18. "Gaps Found in Care, Safety in Mass. Group Homes." *Joint Investigation of the New England Center for Investigative Reporting and WBUR.*

Becker, Gary S., and Murphy, Kevin M. 2013. "Have We Lost the War on Drugs?" *Wall Street Journal.* January 4.

Bell, Kirsten, and Salmon, Amy. 2009. Pain, Physical Dependence, and Pseudoaddiction: Redefining Addiction for 'Nice' People? *International Journal of Drug Policy* 20:170–178.

Berenson, David. 1991. "Powerlessness—Liberating or Enslaving? Responding to the Feminist Critique of the Twelve Steps." Pp. 67–84 in *Feminism and Addiction.* Ed. Claudia Bepko. Binghamton, NY: Haworth Press

Bickel, Christopher. 2010. "From Child to Captive: Constructing Captivity in a Juvenile Institution." *Western Criminology Review* 11(1):37–49.

Binswanger, Ingrid A., Krueger, Patrick M., and Steiner, John F. 2009. "Prevalence of Chronic Medical Conditions among Jail and Prison Inmates in the USA Compared with the General Population." *Journal of Epidemiology and Community Health* 63(11):912–919.

Binswanger, Ingrid A., Stern, Mark F., Deyo, Richard A., Heagerty, Patrick J., Cheadle, Allen, Elmore, Joann G., and Koepsell, Thomas D. 2007. "Release from Prison—A High Risk of Death for Former Inmates." *New England Journal of Medicine* 356:157–165.

Black, M. C., Basile, K. C., Breiding, M. J., Smith, S. G., Walters, M. L., Merrick, M. T., Chen, J., and Stevens, M. R. 2011. *The National Intimate Partner and Sexual Violence Survey (NISVS): 2010 Summary Report.* Atlanta: National Center for Injury Prevention and Control, Centers for Disease Control and Prevention.

Blackburn, Ashley, Mullings, Janet, and Marquart, James W. 2007. "Sexual Assault in Prison and Beyond: Toward an Understanding of Lifetime Sexual Assault among Incarcerated Women." *Prison Journal* 88(3):351–377.

Blackwell, Marilyn. 1999. "The Deserving Sick: Poor Women and the Medicalization of Poverty in Brattleboro, Vermont." *Journal of Women's History* 11(1):53–74.

Blankenship, Kim M., Smoyer, Amy B., Bray, Sarah J., and Mattocks, Kristin. 2005. "Black-White Disparities in HIV/AIDS: The Role of Drug Policy and the Corrections System." *Journal of Health Care for the Poor and Underserved* 16(4 Supp. B):140–158.

Bloom, Barbara, Owen, Barbara, and Covington, Stephanie. 2004. "Women Offenders and the Gendered Effects of Public Policy." *Review of Policy Research* 21(1):31–48.

Boddy, Janice. 1988. "Spirits and Selves in Northern Sudan: The Cultural Therapeutics of Possession and Trance." *American Ethnologist* 15(1):4–27.

Bonilla-Silva, Eduardo. 2013. *Racism without Racists: Color-Blind Racism and the Persistence of Racial Inequality in America.* 4th edition. Lanham, MD: Rowman and Littlefield.

Boston Rental Exchange. 2010. *Boston Rental Facts: The Truth about the Boston Rental Market.* Retrieved from http://www.bostonrentalexchange.com/rental_facts.htm.

Boston Women's Health Book Collective. 2011. *Our Bodies, Ourselves.* 11th ed. New York: Simon and Schuster.

Branson, Richard. 2012. "War on Drugs a Trillion-Dollar Failure." CNN. December 12. Retrieved from http://www.cnn.com/2012/12/06/opinion/branson-end-war-on-drugs/.

Braveman, Paula A., Cubbin, Catherine, Egerter, Susan, Williams, David R. & Pamuk, Elsie. 2010. "Socioeconomic Disparities in Health in the United States." *American Journal of Public Health*, 100(S1):S186–S196.

Britton, Dana M. 2003. *At Work in the Iron Cage: The Prison as Gendered Organization.* New York: New York University Press.

Brook, Kerwin Kaye. 2010. "*Drug Courts and the Treatment of Addiction: Therapeutic Jurisprudence and Neoliberal Governance.*" Ph.D. dissertation, New York University.

Brown, Mildred L., and Rounsley, Chloe Ann. *True Selves: Understanding Transsexualism; for Families, Friends, Coworkers, and Helping Professionals.* San Francisco: Jossey-Bass, 1996.

Brownmiller, Susan. 1975. *Against Our Will: Men, Women and Rape.* New York: Simon and Schuster.

Buchanan, Kim Shayo. 2007. "Impunity: Sexual Abuse in Women's Prisons." *Harvard Civil Rights–Civil Liberties Law Review* 42:45–87.

Bullard, Robert D. 1994. "Poverty, Pollution, and Environmental Racism: Strategies for Building Healthy and Sustainable Communities." Environmental Justice Resource Center. Retrieved from http://www.ejrc.cau.edu/PovpolEj.html.

Bumiller, Kristin. 2008. *In an Abusive State: How Neoliberalism Appropriated the Feminist Movement against Sexual Violence.* Durham, NC: Duke University Press.

Bureau of Labor Statistics. 2011. "Characteristics of Minimum Wage Workers." *Labor Force Statistics from the Current Population Survey: 2011.* Retrieved from http://www.bls.gov/cps/minwage2011.htm.

Bureau of Labor Statistics. 2013. "Usual Weekly Earnings of Wage and Salary Workers, Fourth Quarter, 2012." *U.S. Department of Labor News Release.* Retrieved from http://www.bls.gov/news.release/archives/wkyeng_01182013.pdf.

Bureau of Justice Statistics. 2013. *Prisoners in 2012: Advance Counts.* July 25. Washington, DC: Bureau of Justice Statistics, Office of Justice Programs, U.S. Department of Justice. Retrieved from http://www.bjs.gov.

Butcher, Kristin F., and LaLonde, Robert J. 2006. "Female Offenders Use of Social Welfare Programs before and after Jail and Prison: Does Prison Cause Welfare Dependency?" Federal Reserve Bank of Chicago. Retrieved from http://www.chicagofed.org/digital_assets/publications/working_papers/2006/wp2006_13.pdf.

Cahn, Peter S. 2005. "Saints with Glasses: Mexican Catholics in Alcoholics Anonymous." *Journal of Contemporary Religion* 20(2):217–229.

Callahan, Daniel. 1998. *False Hopes: Why America's Quest for Perfect Health Is a Recipe for Disaster.* New York: Simon and Schuster.

Campbell, Rebecca, and Bybee, Deborah. 1997. "Emergency Medical Services for Rape Victims: Detecting the Cracks in Service Delivery." *Women's Health* 3(2):75–101.

Canfield, Marta C. 2010. "Prescription Opioid Use among Patients Seeking Treatment for Opioid Dependence." *Journal of Addiction Medicine* 4(2): 108–113.

Carr, E. Summerson. 2011. *Scripting Addiction: The Politics of Therapeutic Talk and American Sobriety.* Princeton: Princeton University Press.

Carson, E. Ann, and Golinelli, Daniela. 2013. "Prisoners in 2012: Trends in Admissions and Releases, 1991–2012." Bureau of Justice Statistics, Office of Justice Programs, U.S. Department of Justice. December 19. Retrieved from http://www.bjs.gov /index.cfm?ty=pbdetail&iid=4842.

Cauthen, Nancy K. 2011. "Scheduling Hourly Workers: How Last-Minute, Just-in-Time Scheduling Practices Are Bad for Workers, Families, and Business." *Demos.* Retrieved from http://www.demos.org/sites/default/files/publications/Scheduling_Hourly_Workers_Demos.pdf.

CDC (Centers for Disease Control and Prevention). 2011a. Births—Method of Delivery, 2011. Retrieved from http://www.cdc.gov/nchs/fastats/delivery.htm.

CDC (Centers for Disease Control and Prevention). 2011b. "CDC Health Disparities and Inequalities Report—United States, 2011." *Morbidity and Mortality Weekly Report* 60. Retrieved from http://www.cdc.gov/mmwr/pdf/other/su6001.pdf.

Cecere, David. 2009. "Inmates Suffer from Chronic Illness, Poor Access to Health Care." *Harvard Gazette* (January 15). Retrieved from http://news.harvard.edu /gazette/story/2009/01/inmates-suffer-from-chronic-illness-poor-access-to-health-care/.

Center for Reproductive Rights. 2010. *Reproductive Rights Violations as Torture and Cruel, Inhuman, or Degrading Treatment or Punishment: A Critical Human Rights Analysis.* Retrieved from http://reproductiverights.org/sites/crr.civicactions.net /files/documents/TCIDT.pdf.

Center on Budget and Policy Priorities. 2011. "United States TANF Spending Factsheet." National Poverty Center. Retrieved from http://npc.umich.edu/news /events/safetynet/tanf-spending-factsheet.pdf.

Chadwick, Ben, Waller, Derek G., and Edwards, J. Guy. 2005. "Potentially Hazardous Drug Interactions with Psychotropics." *Advances in Psychiatric Treatment* 11:440–449.

Chapman, Cole. 2013. "A Deadly Trend: Experts Urge Alternative Therapy, Other Ideas to Cut Overdose Numbers." *Sun Chronicle.* July 7. Retrieved from http:// www.thesunchronicle.com/news/local_news/a-deadly-trend/article_3ffd96ee-6655–5701–829c-0581875e2309.html.

Chappell, Allison T. 2013. "Exceptions to the Rule? Exploring the Use of Overrides in Detention Risk Assessment." *Youth Violence and Juvenile Justice* 11(2):332–348.

Charmaz, Kathy. 1999. Stories of Suffering: Subjective Tales and Research Narratives. *Qualitative Health Research* 9(3):362–382.

Chen, Chuan-Yu, and Lin, Keh-Ming. 2009. "Health Consequences of Illegal Drug Use." *Current Opinion in Psychiatry* 22(3):287–292.

Chesney-Lind, Meda. 2002. "Imprisoning Women: The Unintended Victims of Mass Imprisonment." Pp. 79–94 in *Invisible Punishment: The Collateral Consequences of Mass Imprisonment.* Ed. Marc Mauer and Meda Chesney-Lind. New York: The New Press.

Chesney-Lind, Meda, and Pasko, Linda. 2004. *The Female Offender: Girls, Women, and Crime.* 2nd ed. Thousand Oaks, CA: Sage.

Chesney-Lind, Meda, and Eliason, Michele. 2006. "From Invisible to Incorrigible: The Demonization of Marginalized Women and Girls." *Crime, Media, Culture* 2(29): 29–47.

Childbirth Connection. 2013. "Cesarean Section." Retrieved from http://www .childbirthconnection.org.

Child Welfare Information Services. 2008. "Long-Term Consequences of Child Abuse and Neglect." Administration for Children and Families, U.S. Department of Health and Human Services. Retrieved from https://www.childwelfare.gov/pubs /factsheets/long_term_consequences.cfm.

Chopp, Rebecca S. 1986. *The Praxis of Suffering: An Interpretation of Liberation and Political Theologies.* Maryknoll, NY: Orbis Books.

Coffey, Carolyn, Veit, Friederike, Wolfe, Rory, Cini, Eileen, and Patton, George C. 2003. "Mortality in Young Offenders: Retrospective Cohort Study." *British Medical Journal* 326(7398):1064.

Coker, Ann L., Williams, Corrine M., Follingstad, Diane R., and Jordan, Carol E. 2011. "Psychological, Reproductive and Maternal Health, Behavioral, and Economic Impact of Intimate Partner Violence." Pp. 265–284 in *Violence against Women and Children,* Volume 2: *Navigating Solutions.* Ed. Jacquelyn W. White, Mary P. Koss, and Alan E. Kazdin. Washington, DC: American Psychological Association.

Cole, Alyson M. 1999. "'There Are No Victims in This Class': On Female Suffering and Anti-'Victim Feminism.'" *NWSA Journal* 11(1):72–96 (accession no. 1964967).

Cole, Alyson M. 2007. *The Cult of True Victimhood: From the War on Welfare to the War on Terror.* Stanford: Stanford University Press

Collins, Patricia Hill. 2000. *Black Feminist Thought: Knowledge, Consciousness, and the Politics of Empowerment,* 2nd ed. New York: Routledge.

Comfort, Megan. 2007. "Punishment beyond the Legal Offender." *Annual Review of Law and Social Science* 3:271–296.

Connolly, Deborah R. 2000. *Homeless Mothers: Face to Face with Women and Poverty.* Minneapolis: University of Minnesota Press.

Conrad, Peter. 1992. "Medicalization and Social Control." *Annual Review of Sociology* 18:209–232.

Conrad, Peter, and Schneider, Joseph W. 1980. *Deviance and Medicalization: From Badness to Sickness.* St. Louis, MO: Mosby.

Courtenay, Will H. 2011. *Dying to Be Men: Psychosocial, Environmental, and Biobehavioral Directions in Promoting the Health of Men and Boys.* New York: Routledge.

Costa Vargas, Joao H. 2006. *Catching Hell in the City of Angels: Life and Meanings of Blackness in South Central Los Angeles.* Minneapolis: University of Minnesota Press.

Crawford, Robert. 2006. "Health as a Meaningful Social Practice." *Health: An Interdisciplinary Journal for the Social Study of Health, Illness and Medicine* 10(4):401–420.

Crawford Sullivan, Susan. 2011. *Living Faith: Everyday Religion and Mothers in Poverty.* Chicago: University of Chicago Press.

Crenshaw, Kimberlé. 1991. "Mapping the Margins: Intersectionality, Identity Politics, and Violence against Women of Color." *Stanford Law Review* 43(6):1241–1299.

Culhane, Jennifer, Webb, David, Grim, Susan, Metraux, Stephen, and Culhane, Dennis P. 2003. "Prevalence of Child Welfare Service Involvement among Homeless and Low-Income Mothers: A Five-Year Birth Cohort Study." *Journal of Sociology and Social Welfare* 30(3):79–95.

Dáil, Paula vW. 2012. *Women and Poverty in 21st Century America.* Jefferson, NC: McFarland.

Das, Veena. 2010. "Suffering, Theodicies, Disciplinary Practices, Appropriations." *International Social Science Journal* 49(154):563–572.

Davis, Angela Y. 1981. *Women, Race and Class.* NY: Vintage.

Davis, Angela Y., and Shaylor, Cassandra. 2001. "Race, Gender, and the Prison Industrial Complex: California and Beyond." *Meridians* 2(1):1–25.

Davis, Gary L. 2002. "Hepatitis C Interferon Treatment." American Liver Foundation. Retrieved from http://www.interferon.ws/interferon-treatment.htm.

Davis, Robert C., Weisburd, David, and Hamilton, Edwin E. 2010. "Preventing Repeat Incidents of Family Violence: A Randomized Field Test of a Second Responder Program." *Journal of Experimental Criminology* 6(4):397–418.

Decker, Michele R., Erin Pearson, Samantha Illangaselcare, Erin Clark, and Susan G. Sherman. 2013. "Violence against Women in Sex Work and HIV Risk Implications Differ Qualitatively by Perpetrator." *BMC Public Health* (1471–2458) 13(1):876. Accessed online: http://www.biomedcentral.com/1471-2458/13/876

Declercq, Eugene, Cunningham, Deborah K., Johnson, Cynthia and Sakala, Carol. 2008. "Mothers' Reports of Post-Partum Pain Associated with Vaginal and Cesarean Deliveries: Results of a National Survey." *Birth* 35(1):16–24.

DeNavas-Walt, Carmen, Proctor, Bernadette D., Smith, Jessica C. 2013. "Income, Poverty and Health Insurance Coverage in the US: 2012." Current Population Reports, U.S. Census Bureau. Retrieved from http://www.census.gov/newsroom/releases/archives/income_wealth/cb13-165.html.

Desmond, Matthew, and Valdez, Nicol. 2013. "Unpolicing the Urban Poor: Consequences of Third-Party Policing for Inner-City Women." *American Sociological Review* 78:117–141.

Diaz-Cotto, Juanita. 2000. "The Criminal Justice System and Its Impact on Latinas(os) in the United States." *Justice Professional.* 13:49–67.

Dillon, Stephen. 2011. "'The Only Freedom I Can See': Imprisoned Queer Writing and the Politics of the Unimaginable." Pp. 169–184 in *Captive Genders: Trans Embodiment and the Prison Industrial Complex.* Ed. Eric A. Stanley and Nat Smith. Oakland, CA: AK Press.

Dunn, Jennifer L., and Powell-Williams, Melissa. 2007. "'Everybody Makes Choices': Victim Advocates and the Social Construction of Battered Women's Victimization and Agency." *Violence Against Women* 13(10):977–1001.

Eckholm, Erik. 2007. "Disability Cases Last Longer as Backlog Rises." *New York Times.* December 10. Retrieved from http://www.nytimes.com/2007/12/10/us/10disability.html?adxnnl=1&pagewanted=all&adxnnlx=1354302335-jw61XXAroJKPUERd-9cyN8g.

Ezeala-Harrison, Fidel. 2010. "Black Feminization of Poverty: Evidence from the U.S. Cross-Regional Data." *Journal of Developing Areas* 44(1):149.

Farley, Melissa. 2004. "'Bad for the Body, Bad for the Heart': Prostitution Harms Women Even If Legalized or Decriminalized." *Violence Against Women* 10(10):1087–1125.

Fassin, Didier, and Rechtman, Richard. 2009. *The Empire of Trauma: An Inquiry into the Condition of Victimhood*. Princeton: Princeton University Press.

Ferraro, Kathleen J. 2006. *Neither Angels nor Demons: Women, Crime, and Victimization*. Boston: Northeastern University Press.

Ferraro, Kathleen J., and Moe, Angela M. 2003. "Mothering, Crime, and Incarceration." Journal of Contemporary Ethnography 32(1): 9–40.

Finkelhor, David, Turner, Heather, Ormrod, Richard, Hamby, Sherry, and Kracke, Kristin. 2009. "Children's Exposure to Violence: A Comprehensive National Survey." *Juvenile Justice Bulletin* (U.S. Department of Justice, Office of Justice Programs, Office of Juvenile Justice and Delinquency Prevention). Retrieved from http://www.unh.edu/ccrc/pdf/DOJ-NatSCEV-bulletin.pdf.

FitzGerald, Susan G. 2013. "'Crack Baby' Study Ends with Unexpected but Clear Result." *Philadelphia Inquirer*. July 22. Retrieved from http://articles.philly.com/2013-07-22/news/40709969_1_hallam-hurt-so-called-crack-babies-funded-study.

Flanagan, Christine, and Schwartz, Mary. 2013. "Rental Housing Market Condition Measures: A Comparison of U.S. Metropolitan Areas from 2009 to 2011." U.S. Census Bureau. ACSBR/11–07.

Flores, Joan A., and Pellico, Linda H. 2011. "A Meta-synthesis of Women's Postincarceration Experiences." *Journal of Obstetric, Gynecologic, & Neonatal Nursing* 40(4):486–496.

Forman-Hoffman, Valerie L., Zolotor, Adam, McKeeman, Joni L., Blanco, Roberto, Knauer, Stefanie R., Lloyd, Stacey W., Fraser, Jenifer G., and Viswanathan, Meera. 2013. "Comparative Effectiveness of Interventions for Children Exposed to Nonrelational Traumatic Events." *Pediatrics* 131(3):526–539.

Formisano, Ronald P. 1991. *Boston against Busing: Race, Class, and Ethnicity in the 1960s and 1970s*. Chapel Hill: University of North Carolina Press.

Foucault, Michel. 1975. *Discipline and Punish: The Birth of the Prison*. New York: Random House.

Frieden, Thomas, Degutis, Linda, and Spivak, Howard. 2010. "National Intimate Partner and Sexual Violence Survey 2010 Summary Report." Centers for Disease Control and Prevention. Retrieved from http://www.cdc.gov/violenceprevention/pdf/nisvs_report2010-a.pdf.

Fry, Richard, and Taylor, Paul. 2013. "A Rise in Wealth for the Wealthy: Declines for the Lower 93%." Pew Research Center. Retrieved from http://www.pewsocialtrends.org/files/2013/04/wealth_recovery_final.pdf.

Furedi, Frank. 2004. *Therapeutic Culture: Cultivating Vulnerability in an Uncertain Age*. New York: Routledge.

Garcia, Mario, Powers, Kristen, and Hopper, Jessica. 2013. "Prosecutor Leads Effort to Test Long-Abandoned Rape Kits, Brings Justice to Victims." *Rock Center*. February

15. Retrieved from http://rockcenter.nbcnews.com/_news/2013/02/15/15848051-prosecutor-leads-effort-to-test-long-abandoned-rape-kits-brings-justice-to-victims?lite.

Garland, David. 2001. *Mass Imprisonment: Social Causes and Consequences.* London: Sage.

Geertz, Clifford. 1966. "Religion as a Cultural System." Pp. 1–46 in *Anthropological Approaches to the Study of Religion.* Ed. Michael Banton. ASA Monographs 3. London: Tavistock.

Gilens, Martin. 1999. *Why Americans Hate Welfare: Race, Media, and the Politics of Antipoverty Policy.* Studies in Communication, Media and Public Opinion. Chicago: University of Chicago Press.

Glaze, Lauren, and Herberman, Erinn. 2012. "Combined Populations in the US, 2012." Bureau of Justice Statistics, U.S. Department of Justice. Retrieved from http://www.bjs.gov/content/pub/pdf/cpus12.pdf.

Glaze, Lauren E., and Maruschak, Laura M. 2010. "Parents in Prison and Their Minor Children." U.S. Department of Justice, Office of Justice Programs, Bureau of Justice Statistics Special Report. Retrieved from http://www.bjs.gov/content/pub/pdf/pptmc.pdf.

Glaze, Lauren E., and Parks, Erika. 2012. "Correctional Populations in the United States, 2011." U.S. Department of Justice, Office of Justice Programs, Bureau of Justice Statistics (NCJ 239972). Retrieved from http://bjs.gov/content/pub/pdf/cpus11.pdf.

Global Commission on Drug Policy. 2011. *War on Drugs: Report of the Global Commission on Drug Policy.* June. Retrieved from www.globalcommissionondrugs.org.

Glueck, Sheldon, and Glueck, Eleanor Touroff. 1934. *Five Hundred Delinquent Women.* New York: Alfred A. Knopf.

Goffman, Erving. 1961. *Asylums: Essays on the Social Situations of Mental Patients and Other Inmates.* Garden City, NY: Anchor Books.

Gossop, Michael, Stewart, Duncan, and Marsden, John. 2008. "Attendance at Narcotics Anonymous and Alcoholics Anonymous Meetings: Frequency of Attendance and Substance Use Outcome after Residential Treatment for Drug Dependence; a 5-Year Follow-Up Study." *Addiction* 103(1):119–125.

Grant, Jaimie M., Mottet, Lisa A., and Tanis, Justin. 2011. *Injustice at Every Turn: A Report of the National Transgender Discrimination Survey.* Washington, DC: National Center for Transgender Equality and National Gay and Lesbian Task Force.

Greenberg, Gary. 2013. *Book of Woe: The DSM and the Unmaking of Psychiatry.* New York: Blue Rider Press.

Grella, Christine E., Hser, Yih-Ing, and Huang, YuChuang. 2006. "Mothers in Substance Abuse Treatment: Differences in Characteristics Based on Involvement with Child Welfare Services." *Child Abuse and Neglect* 30(1):55–73.

Guerino, Paul, Harrison, Paige M., and Sabol, William J. 2011. "Prisoners in 2010." U.S. Department of Justice, Office of Justice Programs, Bureau of Justice Statistics. Retrieved from: www.bjs.gov/content/pub/pdf/p10.pdf (revised 2/9/12)

Haney, Lynne A. 2010. *Offending Women: Power, Punishment, and the Regulation of Desire*. Berkeley: University of California Press.

Hanley, Michael L. 2008. "A Matter of Racial Justice: The Alarming Disparities of Lead-Poisoning Rates in New York State." *Poverty and Race* 17(1). Retrieved from http://prrac.org.

Harris-Perry, Melissa V. 2011. *Sister Citizen: Shame, Stereotypes, and Black Women in America*. Ann Arbor, MI: Sheridan Books.

Hart, Carl. 2013. *High Price: A Neuroscientist's Journey of Self-Discovery That Challenges Everything You Know about Drugs and Society*. New York: HarperCollins.

Harvey, Mary. 2007. "Towards an Ecological Understanding of Resilience in Trauma Survivors: Implications for Theory, Research, and Practice." *Journal of Aggression, Maltreatment & Trauma* 14(1–2):9–32.

Hasin, Deborah S. et al. 2007. "Prevalence, Correlates, Disability, and Comorbidity of DSM-IV Alcohol Abuse and Dependence in the United States." *Archives of General Psychiatry* 64(7):830–842.

Hausmann, Ricardo, Tyson, Laura D., and Zahidi, Saadia. 2012. *The Global Gender Gap Report, 2012*." Geneva, Switzerland: World Economic Forum. Retrieved from http://www.weforum.org/issues/global-gender-gap.

Hawdon, James E. 2001. "The Role of Presidential Rhetoric in the Creation of a Moral Panic: Reagan, Bush, and the War on Drugs." *Deviant Behavior: An Interdisciplinary Journal* 22:419–445.

Hay, M. Cameron. 2010. "Suffering in a Productive World: Chronic Illness, Visibility, and the Space beyond Agency." *American Ethnologist* 37(2):259–274.

Hays, Sharon. 2003. *Flat Broke with Children: Women in the Age of Welfare Reform*. New York: Oxford University Press.

Heimer, Karen, Johnson, Kecia R., Lang, Joseph B., Rengifo, Andres, F. and Stemen, Don. 2012. "Race and Women's Imprisonment: Poverty, African American Presence, and Social Welfare." *Journal of Quantitative Criminology* 28(2): 219–244.

Henrichson, Christian, and Delaney, Ruth. 2012. *The Price of Prisons: What Incarceration Costs Taxpayers*. Vera Institute of Justice. http://www.vera.org/pubs/special /price-prisons-what-incarceration-costs-taxpayers.

Herman, Judith. 1997. *Trauma and Recovery: The Aftermath of Violence—From Domestic Abuse to Political Terror*. New York: Basic Books.

Herndon, Sharon L. 2001. "The Paradox of Powerlessness: Gender, Sex and Power in 12-Step Groups." *Women and Language* 24(2):7–12.

Herrera, Veronica M., and McCloskey, Laura Ann. 2001. "Gender Differences in the Risk for Delinquency among Youth Exposed to Family Violence." *Child Abuse and Neglect* 25:1037–1052.

Homelessness Research Institute. 2012. "The State of Homelessness in America 2012." National Alliance to End Homelessness. Retrieved from http://b.3cdn.net /naeh/9892745b6de8a5ef59_q2m6yc53b.pdf.

Hopper, Kim, Jost, John, Hay, Terri, Welber, S., and Haugland, Gary. 1997. "Homelessness, Severe Mental Illness, and the Institutional Circuit." *Psychiatry Services* 48(5):659–665.

Horwitz, Allan V., and Wakefield, Jerome C. 2007. *The Loss of Sadness: How Psychiatry Transformed Normal Sorrow into Depressive Disorder.* New York: Oxford University Press.

Humphries, Drew. 1999. *Crack Mothers: Pregnancy, Drugs, and the Media.* Columbus: Ohio State University Press.

Hunnicutt, Gwen. 2009. "Varieties of Patriarchy and Violence against Women: Resurrecting 'Patriarchy' as a Theoretical Tool." *Violence Against Women* 15(5): 553–573.

Iguchi, Martin Y., Bell, James, Ramchand, Rajeev N., and Fain, Terry. 2005. "How Criminal System Racial Disparities May Translate into Health Disparities." *Journal of Health Care for the Poor and Underserved* 16(4):48–56.

Iguchi, Martin Y., London, Jennifer A., Forge, Nell Griffith, Hickman, Laura J., Fain, Terry, and Riechman, Kara. 2002. "Elements of Well-Being Affected by Criminalizing the Drug User." *Public Health Reports* 117(1):146–150. Retrieved from http://www.ncbi.nlm.nih.gov/pmc/articles/PMC1913697/.

Insel, Thomas. 2013. "Director's Blog: Transforming Diagnosis." National Institute of Mental Health. April 29. Retrieved from http://www.nimh.nih.gov/about/director/2013/transforming-diagnosis.shtml.

Irvine, Leslie. 1999. *Codependent Forevermore: The Invention of Self in a Twelve Step Group.* Chicago: University of Chicago Press.

Iyengar, Radha. 2007. "Does the Certainty of Arrest Reduce Domestic Violence? Evidence from Mandatory and Recommended Arrest Laws." National Bureau of Economic Research. Retrieved from http://www.nber.org/papers/w13186.pdf?new_window=1

Jacobson, Margaret, and Occhino, Filippo. 2012. "Labor's Declining Share of Income and Rising Inequality." *Economic Commentary.* Federal Reserve Bank of Cleveland. Retrieved from http://www.clevelandfed.org/research/commentary/2012/2012–13.cfm.

James, Doris J., and Glaze, Lauren E. 2006. *Mental Health Problems of Prison and Jail Inmates.* Bureau of Justice Statistics, Special Report NCJ 213600. Washington, DC: Department of Justice. Retrieved from http://bjs.ojp.usdoj.gov/content/pub/pdf/mhppji.pdf.

Jasinski, Jana L., Wesely, Jennifer K., Wright, James D., and Mustaine, Elizabeth E. 2010. *Hard Lives, Mean Streets: Violence in the Lives of Homeless Women.* Lebanon, NH: Northeastern University Press.

Joffe-Walt, Chana. 2013. "Unfit for Work: The Startling Rise of Disability in America." *All Things Considered.* Nation Public Radio. Broadcast March 22–29. Retrieved from http://apps.npr.org/unfit-for-work/.

Johnson, Byron R. 2002. *Objective Hope: Assessing the Effectiveness of Faith-Based Organizations; A Review of the Literature.* Philadelphia: Center for Research on Religion and Urban Civil Society, University of Pennsylvania.

Johnson, Rucker C., and Raphael, Steven. 2009. "The Effects of Male Incarceration Dynamics on Acquired Immune Deficiency Syndrome Infection Rates among African American Women and Men." *Journal of Law and Economics* 52(2):251–293.

Kaminer, Wendy. 1992. *I'm Dysfunctional, You're Dysfunctional: The Recovery Movement and Other Self-Help Fashions.* Reading, MA: Addison-Wesley.

Kaskutas, Lee Ann. 2009. "Alcoholics Anonymous Effectiveness: Faith Meets Science." *Journal of Addictive Diseases* 28(2):145–157.

Kasl, Charlotte D. 1992. *Many Roads, One Journey: Moving beyond the 12 Steps.* New York: Harper Collins.

Kirk, Stuart A., Gomory, Tomi, and Cohen, David. 2013. *Mad Science: Psychiatric Coercion, Diagnosis, and Drugs.* New Brunswick, NJ: Transaction.

Kleinman, Arthur. 1994. "Pain and Resistance: The Delegitimation and Relegitimation of Local Worlds." Pp. 169–197 in *Pain as Human Experience: An Anthropological Perspective.* Ed. Mary-Jo DelVecchio Good, Paul E. Brodwin, Byron J. Good, and Arthur Kleinman. Berkeley: University of California Press.

Koss, Mary. 2006. "Restoring Rape Survivors: Justice, Advocacy and a Call to Action." *Violence and Exploitation against Women and Girls* 1087:206–234.

Kozol, Johnathan. 1985. *Death at an Early Age.* New York: Penguin Group.

Kronstadt, Jessica. 2008. "Health and Economic Mobility." The Urban Institute. Retrieved from http://www.urban.org/UploadedPDF/1001161_Health.pdf.

Lasser, Karen E., Kronman, Andrea C., Cabral, Howard, and Samet, Jeffrey H. 2012. "Emergency Department Use by Primary Care Patients at a Safety-Net Hospital." *Archives of Internal Medicine* 172(3):278–280.

Latin American Herald Tribune. 2013. "Drug Cartels Make $64 Billion a Year from U.S., Mexican Says." Retrieved from http://www.laht.com/article.asp?ArticleId= 342471&CategoryId=14091.

LaVene, Meredith C., White, Mary C., Waters, Catherine M., and Tulsky, Jacqueline P. 2003. "Screening for Health Conditions in a County Jail: Differences by Gender." *Journal of Correctional Health Care* 9(4):381–396.

Lee, Suevon. 2012. "By the Numbers: The U.S.'s Growing For-Profit Detention Industry." *ProPublica: Journalism in the Public Interest.* Retrieved from http://www.propublica. org/article/by-the-numbers-the-u.s.s-growing-for-profit-detention-industry.

Leonard, Elizabeth Dermody. 2002. *Convicted Survivors.* SUNY Series in Women, Crime, and Criminology. Albany: State University of New York Press.

Lester, Rebecca J. 1999. "Let Go and Let God: Religion and the Politics of Surrender in Overeaters Anonymous." Pp. 139–164 in *Interpreting Weight: The Social Management of Fatness and Thinness.* Ed. Jeffery Sobal and Donna Maurer. New York: Aldine de Gruyter.

Lester, Rebecca J. 2011. "Local Responses to Trauma and PTSD: Discussant Comments." Paper presented at the American Anthropological Association Annual Meeting, Montreal, November 16.

Leverentz, Andrea M. 2014. *The Ex-Prisoner's Dilemma: How Women Negotiate Competing Narratives of Reentry and Desistance.* New Brunswick, NJ: Rutgers University Press.

Lichtenwalter, Sara. 2005. "Gender Poverty Disparity in U.S. Cities: Evidence Exonerating Female-Headed Families." *Journal of Sociology and Social Welfare* 32(2):75–96.

Lipsitz, George. 2012. "In an Avalanche Every Snowflake Pleads Not Guilty: The Collateral Consequences of Mass Incarceration and Impediments to Women's Fair Housing Rights." *UCLA Law Review* 59(6):1746–1809.

Lundström, B., and Wålinder, Pauly J. 2007. "Outcome of Sex Reassignment Surgery." *Acta Psychiatrica Scandinavica* 70(4):289–294.

Macartney, Suzanne, Bishaw, Alemayehu, and Fontenot, Kayla. 2013. *Poverty Rates for Selected Detailed Race and Hispanic Groups by State and Place, 2007–2011.* American Community Survey Briefs. Washington, DC: U.S. Census Bureau.

MacDorman, Marian F., and Mathews, T. J. 2011. "Understanding Racial and Ethnic Disparities in U.S. Infant Mortality Rates." NCHS Data Brief 74. National Center for Health Statistics, Centers for Disease Control and Prevention. http://www.cdc.gov/nchs/data/databriefs/db74.htm.

Maher, Lisa. 2000. *Sexed Work: Gender, Race, and Resistance in a Brooklyn Drug Market.* New York: Oxford University Press.

Mallicoat, Stacy. 2007. "Gendered Justice Attributional Differences between Males and Females in the Juvenile Courts." *Feminist Criminology* 2(1):4–30.

Mallik-Kane, Kamala, and Visher, Christy A. 2008. *Health and Prisoner Reentry: How Physical, Mental, and Substance Abuse Conditions Shape the Process of Reintegration.* Washington, DC: Urban Institute Justice Policy Center.

Mangano, Philip. 2007. "High Users of Publicly-Funded Health Services: A Strategy for Reducing Spending While Improving Care" (United States Interagency Council on Homelessness). Paper presented at Common Ground–NASHP meeting, April 24–25, New York City.

Manza, Jeff, and Uggen, Christopher. 2008. *Locked Out: Felon Disenfranchisement and American Democracy.* Oxford: Oxford University Press.

Marmot, Michael, and Wilkinson, Richard G. 2006. *Social Determinants of Health.* Oxford: Oxford University Press.

Martin, Laura, Hearst, Mary O., and Widome, Rachel. 2010. "Meaningful Differences: Comparison of Adult Women Who First Traded Sex as a Juvenile versus as an Adult." *Violence Against Women* 16(11):1252–1269.

Martin, Sandra L., Macy, Rebecca J., and Young, Siobhan K. 2011. "Health and Consequences of Sexual Violence." Pp. 173–195 in *Violence against Women and Children, Volume 1: Mapping the Terrain.* Ed. Jacqueline W. White, Mary P. Koss, and Alan E. Kazdin. Washington, DC: American Psychological Association.

Mason, Cody. 2012. *Too Good to Be True: Private Prisons in America.* Washington, DC: Sentencing Project.

Massachusetts Department of Corrections. 2008. "January 1, 2008, Population Statistics." Publication 08–122–02 Doc. May. Retrieved from http://www.mass.gov/doc.

Massachusetts Department of Corrections. 2013. "Prison Population Trends." Retrieved from http://www.mass.gov/eopss/docs/doc/research-reports/pop-trends/prisonpoptrendsfinal-2012.pdf.

Massachusetts Executive Office of Public Safety and Security. 2013. "Frequently Asked Question about the DOC." Retrieved from http://www.mass.gov/eopss/agencies/doc/faqs-about-the-doc.html.

Massoglia, Michael. 2008a. "Incarceration as Exposure: The Prison, Infectious Disease, and Other Stress Related Illnesses." *Journal of Health and Social Behavior* 49(1):56–71.

Massoglia, Michael. 2008b. "Incarceration, Health and Racial Disparities in Health." *Law & Society Review* 42(2):275–306.

Massoglia, Michael, Pare, Paul-Philippe, Schnittker, Jason, and Gagnon, Alain. 2014. "The Relationship between Incarceration and Premature Adult Mortality: Gender Specific Evidence." Social Science Research 46:142–154.

Mathieu, Arline. 1993. "The Medicalization of Homelessness and the Theater of Repression." *Medical Anthropology Quarterly* 7(2):170–184.

Mauer, Marc. 2006. *Race to Incarcerate*. New York: The New Press.

Mauer, Marc. 2013. "The Changing Racial Dynamics." The Sentencing Project. Retrieved from http://www.sentencingproject.org/detail/publication.cfm?publication_id=432&id=136.

McCay, Vernon. 1995. "ADA and the Hearing Impaired: New Rights for Inmates with Hearing Loss." *Corrections Today* 57:140.

McCorkel, Jill A. 2013. *Breaking Women: Gender, Race, and the New Politics of Imprisonment*. New York: New York University Press.

McDaniels-Wilson, Cathy, and Belknap, Joanne. 2008. "The Extensive Sexual Violation and Sexual Abuse Histories of Incarcerated Women." *Violence Against Women* 14(10):1090–1127.

McKim, Allison. 2008. "'Getting Gut-Level': Punishment, Gender, and Therapeutic Governance." *Gender & Society* 22(3):303–323.

McFarland, Michael J. 2009. "Religion and Mental Health among Older Adults: Do the Effects of Religious Involvement Vary by Gender?" *Journal of Gerontology* 65B(5):621–630.

McLaughlin, P. J. 2008. *January 1, 2008, Inmate Statistics*. Concord: Research and Planning Division, Massachusetts Department of Correction. Retrieved from http://www.mass.gov/eopss/docs/doc/research-reports/jan-1-population/112008.pdf.

Mercadante, Linda A. 1996. *Victims and Sinners: Spiritual Roots of Addiction and Recovery*. Louisville, KY: Westminster John Knox Press.

Messina, N., and Grella, C. 2006. "Childhood Trauma and Women's Health Outcomes in a California Prison Population." *American Journal of Public Health* 96(10):1842–1848.

Metzner, Jeffrey L., and Fellner, Jamie. 2010. "Solitary Confinement and Mental Illness in US Prisons: A Challenge for Medical Ethics." *Journal of the American Academy of Psychiatry and the Law* 38:104–108.

Mukherjee, D. V., et al. 2013. "Prevalence and Risk Factors for *Staphylococcus aureus* Colonization in Individuals Entering Maximum-Security Prisons." *Epidemiology and Infection* 0950–2688:1–10.

Miller, Eric J. 2004. "Embracing Addiction: Drug Courts and the False Promise of Judicial Interventionism." *Ohio State Law Journal* 65: 1479–1576.

Mills, Linda G. 2003. *Insult to Injury: Rethinking Our Responses to Intimate Abuse.* Princeton: Princeton University Press.

Mogul, Joey L., Ritchie, Andrea J., and Whitlock, Kay. 2011. *Queer (In)justice: The Criminalization of LGBT People in the United States.* Boston: Beacon Press.

Morone, James A. 2009. "Jefferson's Rickety Wall: Sacred and Secular in American Politics." *Social Research* 74(4):1199–1226.

Morris, David B. 1991. *The Culture of Pain.* Berkeley: University of California Press.

Mulia, Nina. 2002. "Ironies in the Pursuit of Well-Being: The Perspectives of Low-Income, Substance-Using Women on Service Institutions." *Contemporary Drug Problems* 29:711–748.

National Center for Chronic Disease Prevention and Health Promotion. 2009. *What Work?* Department of Health and Human Services and Centers for Disease Control and Prevention. Retrieved from: www.cdc.gov/chronicdisease/resources/publications/aag/chronic.htm

National Coalition for the Homeless. 2009. "Health Care and Homelessness." Factsheet. Retrieved from http://www.nationalhomeless.org/factsheets/health.html.

National Commission on Correctional Health Care. 2002. "The Health Status of Soon-to-Be-Released Inmates: A Report to Congress." Volume 1. March. Retrieved from https://www.ncjrs.gov/pdffiles1/nij/grants/189735.pdf.

National Institute of Justice. 2011. "Drug Courts." Retrieved from http://www.nij.gov/topics/courts/drug-courts/Pages/welcome.aspx.

National Institute on Alcohol Abuse and Alcoholism. 2014. Alcohol Facts and Statistics. Retrieved from http://www.niaaa.nih.gov/alcohol-health/overview-alcohol-consumption/alcohol-facts-and-statistics.

National Institute on Drug Abuse. (2011). *Topics in Brief: Prescription Drug Abuse.* Retrieved from http://www.drugabuse.gov/publications/topics-in-brief/prescription-drug-abuse.

National Law Center on Homelessness and Poverty. (2007). *Lost Housing, Lost Safety: Survivors of Domestic Violence Experience Housing Denials and Evictions across the Country.* Retrieved from http://www.nlchp.org/content/pubs/NNEDV-NLCHP_Joint_Stories%20_February_20072.pdf.

Nedderman, A. Barbara, Underwood, Lee A., and Hardy, Veronica L. 2010. "Spirituality Group with Female Prisoners: Impacting Hope." *Journal of Correctional Health Care* 16(2):117–132.

Nevin, Rick. 2007. "Understanding International Crime Trends: The Legacy of Pre-School Lead Exposure." *Environmental Research* 104:315–336.

Nieto, Marcus. 2002. "In Danger of Falling through the Cracks: Children of Arrested Parents." California Research Bureau. Retrieved from http://www.library.ca.gov/crb/02/09/02-009.pdf.

Nixon, Kendra L., Tutty, Leslie M., Downe, Pamela, Gorkoff, Kelly, and Ursal, E. Jone. 2002. "The Everyday Occurrence: Violence in the Lives of Girls Exploited through Prostitution." *Violence Against Women* (8):1016–1043.

Norton-Hawk, Maureen, Sered, Susan, and Mastrorilli, Mary Ellen. 2013. "History Repeats Itself: The Life Course of Women Released from Prison." *Offender Programs Report* 17(3):35–36.

O'Connell, James J. 2005. *Premature Mortality in Homeless Populations: A Review of the Literature.* Nashville: National Health Care for the Homeless Council, December. Retrieved from http://santabarbarastreetmedicine.org/wordpress/wp-content /uploads/2011/04/PrematureMortalityFinal.pdf.

U.S. Office of Family Assistance. 2012. "Characteristics and Financial Circumstances of TANF Recipients, Fiscal Year 2010." U.S. Department of Health, Administration for Children and Families. Retrieved from http://www.acf.hhs.gov/programs/ofa /resource/character/fy2010/fy2010chap10-ys-final.

Olshansky, S. Jay, Antonucci, Toni, Berkman, Lisa, Binstock, Robert H., Boersch-Supan, Axel, Cacioppo, John T., Carnes, Bruce A., Carstensen, Laura L., Fried, Linda P., Goldman, Dana P., Jackson, James, Kohli, Martin, Rother, John, Zheng, Yuhui, and Rowe, John. 2012. "Differences in Life Expectancy Due to Race and Educational Differences Are Widening, and Many May Not Catch Up." *Health Affairs* 31(8):1803–1813.

Osypuk, Theresa L. and Acevedo-Garcia, Dolores. 2010. "Beyond Individual Neighborhoods: A Geography of Opportunity Perspective for Understanding Racial /Ethnic Health Disparities." *Health Place* 16(6):1113–1123.

Owen, Barbara. 1998. *In the Mix: Struggle and Survival in a Women's Prison.* Albany: State University of New York Press.

Pascoe, Elizabeth A., and Richman, Laura Smart. 2009. "Perceived Discrimination and Health: A Meta-analytic Review." *Psychological Bulletin* 135(4):531–554.

Pelissier, Bernadette, and Jones, Nicole. 2006. "Differences in Motivation, Coping Style, and Self-Efficacy among Incarcerated Male and Female Drug Users." *Journal of Substance Abuse and Treatment* 30(2):113–120.

Pew Center on the States. 2011. *State of Recidivism: The Revolving Door of America's Prisons.* Washington, DC: Pew Charitable Trusts.

Pew Charitable Trusts. 2009. "One in 31: The Long Reach of American Corrections." Retrieved from http://www.pewstates.org/uploadedFiles/PCS_Assets/2009/ PSPP_1in31_report_FINAL_WEB_3-26-09.pdf.

Phillips, Susan D. 2013. "Fact Sheet: Parents in State Prisons." The Sentencing Project. Retrieved from http://www.sentencingproject.org/detail/publication .cfm?publication_id=487&id=136.

Phillips, Susan D., Erkanli, Alaattin, Keeler, Gordon P., Costello, E. Jane, and Angold, Adrian. 2006. "Disentangling the Risks: Parent Criminal Justice Involvement and Children's Exposure to Family Risks." *Criminology and Public Policy* 5(4): 677–702.

Political Research Associates. 2005. "Poverty and the Criminal Justice System: Factsheet." *Defending Justice: An Activist Resource Kit.* Retrieved from http://www .publiceye.org/defendingjustice/pdfs/factsheets/11-Fact%20Sheet%20%20Poverty .pdf.

Pollack, Shoshana. 2005. "Taming the Shrew: Regulating Prisoners through Women-Centered Mental Health Programming." *Critical Criminology* 13(1):71–87.

Ptacek, James. 2010. *Restorative Justice and Violence against Women*. New York: Oxford University Press.

Qiuping Gu, Dillon, Charles F., and Burt, Vicki L. 2010. "Prescription Drug Use Continues to Increase: U.S. Prescription Drug Data for 2007–2008." NCHS Data Brief 42. National Center for Health Statistics, Centers for Disease Control and Prevention. Retrieved from http://www.cdc.gov/nchs/data/databriefs/db42.htm.

RAINN (Rape, Abuse & Incest National Network). 2009. *Reporting Rates*. Retrieved from http://www.rainn.org/get-information/statistics/reporting-rates.

Raphael, Jody. 2007. *Freeing Tammy: Women, Drugs, and Incarceration*. Lebanon, NH: Northeastern University Press.

Rathbone, Cristina. 2007. *A World Apart: Women, Prison, and Life behind Bars*. New York: Random House.

Reiman, Amanda. "Moral Philosophy and Social Work Policy." 2009. *Journal of Social Work Values and Ethics* 6(3):136. Retrieved from http://0-www.ncbi.nlm.nih.gov.

Reinarman, Craig, and Levine, Harry G. 1997. *Crack in America: Demon Drugs and Social Justice*. Berkeley: University of California Press.

Research and Planning Division, Massachusetts Department of Correction. 2013. *Prison Population Trends, 2012*. Retrieved from http://www.mass.gov/eopss/docs/doc/research-reports/pop-trends/prisonpoptrendsfinal-2012.pdf.

Richie, Beth E. 1996. *Compelled to Crime: The Gender Entrapment of Battered Black Women*. New York: Routledge.

Richie, Beth E. 2012. *Arrested Justice: Black Women, Violence, and America's Prison Nation*. New York: New York University Press.

Philip Rieff. 1987. *The Triumph of the Therapeutic: Uses of Faith after Freud*. Chicago: University of Chicago Press.

Riger, Stephanie, and Gordon, Margaret. 2010. "The Fear of Rape: A Study in Social Control." *Journal of Social Issues* 37(4):71–92.

Roberts, Dorothy. 1997. *Killing the Black Body*. New York: Random House.

Rochon, Paula, and Gurwitz, Jerry. 1997. "Optimizing Drug Treatment for Elderly People: The Prescribing Cascade." *British Medical Journal* 315(7115):1096–1099.

Rose, Tricia. 2003. *Longing to Tell: Black Women's Stories of Sexuality and Intimacy*. New York: Picador.

Rosen, David L., Schoenbach, Victor J., and Wohl, D.A. 2008. "All-Cause and Cause-Specific Mortality among Men Released from State Prison, 1980–2005." *American Journal of Public Health* 98(12):2278–2284.

Rosenblum, Darren. 1999–2000. "Trapped in Sing Sing: Transgendered Prisoners Caught in the Gender Binarism." *Michigan Journal of Gender & Law* 6:499–572.

Sabo, Don. 2001. "Doing Time, Doing Masculinity: Sports and Prison." Pp. 61–66 in *Prison Masculinities*. Ed. Don Sabo, Terry A. Kupers, and Willie London. Philadelphia: Temples University Press.

Sabo, Don, Kupers, Terry A., and London, Willie (Eds.). 2001. *Prison Masculinities*. Philadelphia: Temple University Press.

Sabol, William J. 2011. "Demographics of the Correctional Population and Implications for Correctional Health Care." Paper presented at the Academic and Health Policy Conference on Correctional Health, University of Massachusetts, Boston.

SAMHSA (Substance Abuse and Mental Health Services Administration). 2012. *Results from the 2011 National Survey on Drug Use and Health: Summary of National Findings*. NSDUH Series H-44, HHS Publication No. (SMA) 12–4713. Rockville, MD: Substance Abuse and Mental Health Services Administration.

SAMHSA (Substance Abuse and Mental Health Services Administration). 2013. *Results from the 2012 National Survey on Drug Use and Health: Summary of National Findings*. NSDUH Series H-46, HHS Publication No. (SMA) 13–4795. Rockville, MD: Substance Abuse and Mental Health Services Administration.

Sanday, Peggy Reeves. 2003. "Rape-Free versus Rape-Prone: How Culture Makes a Difference." Pp. 337–362 in *Evolution, Gender, and Rape*. Ed. Cheryl Brown Travis. Cambridge, MA: MIT Press.

Schmitt, John, Warner, Kris, and Gupta, Sarika. 2010. "The High Budgetary Cost of Incarceration." Center for Economic and Policy Research. Retrieved from http://www.cepr.net/index.php/publications/reports/the-high-budgetary-cost-of-incarceration/.

Schnittker, Jason, and John, Andrea. 2007. "Enduring Stigma: The Long-Term Effects of Incarceration on Health." *Journal of Health and Social Behavior* 48(2):115–130.

Schnittker, Jason, Massoglia, Michael, and Uggen, Christopher. 2012. "Out and Down: Incarceration and Psychiatric Disorders." *Journal of Health and Social Behavior* 53(4):448–464.

Schoenfeld, Heather. 2012. "The War on Drugs, the Politics of Crime, and Mass Incarceration in the United States." *Journal of Gender, Race and Justice* 15(2): 315–352.

Scoular, Jane. 2004. "The 'Subject' of Prostitution: Interpreting the Discursive, Symbolic, and Material Position of Sex/Work in Feminist Theory." *Feminist Theory* 5:343–355.

Scully, Judith A. M. 2002. "Killing the Black Community: A Commentary on the United States War on Drugs." Pp. 55–80 in *Policing the National Body: Race, Gender, and Criminalization*. Ed. Jael Silliman and Anannya Bhattacharjee. Cambridge, MA: South End Press.

Seabrook, Jeremy. 2002. *The No-Nonsense Guide to Class, Caste, and Hierarchies*. London: New Internationalist.

Sered, Susan S. 1994. *Priestess, Mother, Sacred Sister: Religions Dominated by Women*. New York: Oxford University Press.

Sered, Susan S., and Agigian, Amy. 2008. "Holistic Sickening: Breast Cancer and Discursive Worlds of Complementary and Alternative Practitioners." *Sociology of Health and Illness* 30(4):616–31.

Sered, Susan S., and Fernandopulle, Rushika. 2005. *Uninsured in America: Life and Death in the Land of Opportunity*. Berkeley: University of California Press.

Sered, Susan S., and Norton-Hawk, Maureen. 2011a. "Gender Overdetermination and Resistance: The Case of Criminalized Women." *Feminist Theory* 12(3):317–333.

Sered, Susan S., and Norton-Hawk, Maureen. 2011b. "Whose Higher Power: Criminalized Women Confront the Twelve Steps." *Feminist Criminology* 6(4): 308–322.

Sered, Susan S., and Norton-Hawk, Maureen. 2013. "Criminalized Women and the Healthcare System: The Case for Continuity of Services." *Journal of Correctional Health Care* 19(3):164–177.

Sharma, Ursula. 1999. *Caste.* Philadelphia: Open University Press.

Shaylor, Cassandra. 1998. "It's Like Living in a Black Hole: Women of Color and Solitary Confinement in the Prison Industrial Complex." *New England Journal on Criminal and Civil Confinement* 24:385–416.

Smith, Brendan L. 2012. "Inappropriate Prescribing." *Monitor on Psychology* 43(6). Retrieved from https://www.apa.org/monitor/2012/06/prescribing.aspx.

Solnit, Rebecca. 2013. "The Longest War Is the One Against Women." *Common Dreams.* January 24. Retrieved from http://www.tomdispatch.com/post/175641/.

Sontag, Susan. 2003. *Regarding the Pain of Others.* New York: Picador.

Sorenson, Susan, and Garman, Keri. 2013. "How to Tackle U.S. Employees' Stagnating Engagement." *Gallup Business Journal.* Retrieved from http://businessjournal.gallup.com/content/162953/tackle-employees-stagnating-engagement.aspx.

Soss, Joe, Fording, Richard C., and Schram, Sanford F. 2012. *Disciplining the Poor: Neoliberal Paternalism and the Persistent Power of Race.* Chicago: University of Chicago Press.

Stargardter, Gabriel. 2013. "U.N. Development Chief Flags Failures of the War on Drugs." Reuters. March 14. Mexico City. Retrieved from http://www.reuters.com/article/2013/03/14/us-un-drugs-idUSBRE92D12C20130314.

Stone, Deborah A. 1979. "Diagnosis and the Dole: The Function of Illness in American Distributive Politics." *Journal of Health Politics, Policy and Law* 4(3):507–521.

Sudbury, Julia. 2005. "Introduction: Feminist Critiques, Transnational Landscapes, Abolitionist Visions." Pp. xi–xxviii in *Global Lockdown: Race, Gender, and the Prison-Industrial Complex.* Ed. Julia Sudbury. New York: Routledge.

Sullivan, Winnifred F. 2009. *Prison Religion: Faith-Based Reform and the Constitution.* Princeton: Princeton University Press.

Sullivan, Winnifred F. 2010. "Religion Naturalized: The New Establishment." *After Pluralism: Reimaging Religious Engagement.* Eds. Courtney Bender and Pamela Klassen. New York: Columbia University Press.

Swatos, William H. 2006. "Implicit Religious Assumptions within the Resurgence of Civil Religion in the USA since 9/11." *Implicit Religion* 9(2):166–179.

Swendsen Joel, Conway, Kevin P., Degenhardt, Louisa, Glantz, Meyer, Jin, Robert, Merikangas, Kathleen R., Sampson, Nancy, and Kessler, Ronald C. 2010. "Mental Disorders as Risk Factors for Substance Use, Abuse, and Dependence: Results from the 10-Year Follow-Up of the National Comorbidity Survey." *British Journal of Addiction* (0952–0481) 105(6):1117.

Symington, Alison. 2004. "Intersectionality: A Tool for Gender and Economic Justice." *Women's Rights and Economic Change* 9. Retrieved from http://www.awid.org/Library/Intersectionality-A-Tool-for-Gender-and-Economic-Justice2.

Szasz, Thomas. 1992. *Our Right to Drugs: The Case for a Free Market.* New York: Praeger.

Tallen, Bette S. 1990. "Twelve Step Programs: A Lesbian Feminist Critique." *NWSA Journal* 2(3):390–407.

Thomas, James C., and Torrone, Elizabeth. 2006. "Incarceration as Forced Migration: Effects on Selected Community Health Outcomes." *American Journal of Public Health* 96(10):1762–1765.

Thompson, Melissa. 2010. *Mad or Bad: Race, Class, Gender, and Mental Disorder in the Criminal Justice System.* El Paso, TX: LFB Scholarly.

Throop, C. Jason. 2010. *Suffering and Sentiment: Exploring the Vicissitudes of Experience and Pain in Yap.* Berkeley: University of California Press.

Tjaden, Patricia, and Thoennes, Nancy. 1998. *Prevalence, Incidence, and Consequences of Violence against Women: Findings from the National Violence against Women Survey.* Washington, DC: National Institute of Justice and Centers for Disease Control and Prevention.

Tracy, Steven R. 2007. "Patriarchy and Domestic Violence: Challenging Common Misconceptions." *Journal of the Evangelical Theological Society* 50(3):573–594.

Travis, Jeremy, and Waul, Michelle. 2003. *Prisoners Once Removed: The Impact of Incarceration and Reentry on Children, Families, and Communities.* Washington, DC: Urban Institute Press.

Uggen, Christopher, Manza, Jeff, and Thompson, Melissa. 2006. "Citizenship, Democracy, and the Civic Reintegration of Criminal Offenders." *Annals of the American Academy of Political and Social Science* 605:281–310.

Uggen, Christopher, Shannon, Sarah, and Manza, Jeff. 2012. "State-Level Estimates of Felon Disenfranchisement in the United State, 2010." Sentencing Project. August 20. Retrieved from http://www.sentencingproject.org/detail/news.cfm?news_id=1334.

UNODC (United Nations Office on Drugs and Crime). 2011. *Estimating Illicit Financial Flows Resulting from Drug Trafficking.* Research report, October. Vienna: UNODC. Retrieved from http://www.unodc.org/documents/data-and-analysis/Studies/Illicit_financial_flows_2011_web.pdf.

Zedlewski, Sheila. 2012. "Fifteen Years after Welfare Reform Took Hold, How Well Does the Program Work?" Urban Institute. Retrieved from http://www.urban.org/url.cfm?ID=901500&renderforprint=1.

United Nations General Assembly. 1993. "Resolution 48/104 (1993) [Declaration of the Elimination of Violence against Women]" (A/RES/48/104). 85th Plenary Meeting, December 20. Retrieved from http://www.un.org/documents/ga/res/48/a48r104.htm.

U.S. Census Bureau. 2012. *American Community Survey.* Retrieved from https://www.census.gov/newsroom/releases/archives/american_community_survey_acs/cb13-r67.html.

U.S. Conference of Mayors. 2007. "A Status Report on Hunger and Homelessness in America's Cities: A 23-City Survey, December, 2007." *Hunger and Homelessness Survey.* Retrieved from http://usmayors.org/hhsurvey2007/hhsurvey07.pdf.

U.S. Government Accountability Office. 2008. "Young Adults with Serious Mental Illness." June. Retrieved from http://www.gao.gov/products/GAO-08-678.

U.S. Government Accountability Office. 2012. "Children's Mental Health: Concerns Remain about Appropriate Services for Children in Medicaid and Foster Care." Retrieved from http://www.gao.gov/assets/660/650716.pdf.

U.S. Social Security Administration. 2013. *SSI Annual Statistical Report.* December. Retrieved from http://www.ssa.gov/policy/docs/chartbooks/fast_facts/2013/fast_facts13.html#page24.

Van Bruggen, Lisa K., Runtz, Marsha G., and Kadlec, Helena. 2006. "Sexual Revictimization: The Role of Sexual Self-Esteem and Dysfunctional Sexual Behaviors." *Child Maltreatment* 11(2):131–145.

Veysey, Bonita M., Coue, K. D., and Prescott, L. 1998. "Effective Management of Female Jail Detainees with Histories of Physical and Sexual Abuse." *American Jails* 12(2):50–54.

Wacquant, Loic. 2009. *Punishing the Poor: The Neoliberal Government of Social Insecurity.* Durham, NC: Duke University Press.

Ware, Wesley. 2011. "'Rounding Up the Homosexuals': The Impact of Juvenile Court on Queer and Trans/Gender Non-conforming Youth." Pp. 77–84 in *Captive Genders: Trans Embodiment and the Prison Industrial Complex.* Ed. Eric A. Stanley and Nat Smith. Oakland, CA: AK Press.

Watters, Ethan. 2010. *Crazy like Us: The Globalization of the American Psyche.* New York: Free Press.

Weaver, Robert, and Duongtran, Paul. 2009. "Public Perceptions of Parenting and Work Behaviors of Mothers in Receipt of Welfare." *Journal of Policy Practice* 9(1):18–35.

West, Heather C. 2010. "Prison Inmates at Midyear 2009—Statistical Tables." U.S. Department of Justice, Office of Justice Programs, Bureau of Justice Statistics. Retrieved from http://bjs.gov/content/pub/pdf/pim09st.pdf.

Whitaker, Robert. 2010. *Anatomy of an Epidemic: Magic Bullets, Psychiatric Drugs, and the Astonishing Rise of Mental Illness in America.* New York: Broadway Paperbacks.

White, Jacqueline W., Koss, Mary P., and Kazdin, Alan E., Eds. 2011. *Violence against Women and Children, Volume 1: Mapping the Terrain.* Washington, DC: American Psychological Association.

White House Council on Women and Girls. 2012. "Keeping America's Women Moving Forward: The Key to an Economy Built to Last." April. Retrieved from http://m.whitehouse.gov/sites/default/files/email-files/womens_report_final_for_print.pdf.

WHO (World Health Organization). 2013. Trade, Foreign Policy, Diplomacy, and Health: Pharmaceutical Industry. Retrieved from http://www.who.int/trade/glossary/story073/en/.

Wilkinson, Richard, and Pickett, Kate. 2009. *The Spirit Level: Why More Equal Societies Almost Always Do Better*. New York: Bloomsbury Press.

Williams, David R., and Mohammed, Selina A. 2009. "Discrimination and Racial Disparities in Health: Evidence and Needed Research." *Journal of Behavioral Medicine*, 32(1):20–47.

Wilper, Andrew P., Woolhandler, Steffie, Boyd, J. Wesley, Lasser, Karen E., McCormick, Danny, Bor, David H., and Himmelstein, David U. 2009. "The Health and Health Care of US Prisoners: A Nationwide Survey." *American Journal of Public Health* 99(4):1–7.

Wood, Peter B., and May, David C. 2003. "Race Differences in Perceptions of Sanction Severity: A Comparison of Prison with Alternatives." *Justice Quarterly* 20:605–631.

Wu, Shin-Yi, and Green, Anthony. 2000. *Projection of Chronic Illness Prevalence and Cost Inflation*. Santa Monica, CA: RAND Health. Retrieved from http://www.cdc.gov/chronicdisease/overview/index.htm.

Wu, L. T., Woody, G. E., Yang, C., Pan, J. J., Blazer, D. G. 2011. "Racial/Ethnic Variations in Substance-Related Disorders among Adolescents in the United States." *Archives of General Psychiatry* 68:1176–1185.

Xavier, Jessica M. 2000. *The Washington, DC, Transgender Needs Assessment Survey Final Report for Phase Two*. Gender Education and Advocacy, Inc. Retrieved from http://www.gender.org/resources/dge/gea01011.pdf.

Yehuda, Rachel, Pratchett, Laura, and Pelcovitz, Michelle. 2012. "Biological Contributions to PTSD: Differentiating Normative from Pathological Response." Pp. 159–174 in *The Oxford Handbook of Traumatic Stress Disorders*, ed. J. Gayle Beck and Denise M. Sloan. New York: Oxford University Press.

Zaitzow, Barbara H. 2010. "Psychotropic Control of Women Prisoners: The Perpetuation of Abuse of Imprisoned Women." *Justice Policy Journal* 7(2). Retrieved from http://www.cjcj.org/files/Psychotropic_Control.pdf.

Zehr, Howard, and Mika, Harry. 1998. "Fundamental Concepts of Restorative Justice." *Contemporary Justice Review* 1:47–55.

Zito, Julie M., Safer, Daniel J., Sai, Devadatta, Gardner, James F., Thomas, Diane, Coombes, Phyllis, Dubowski, Melissa, and Mendez-Lewis, Maria. 2008. "Psychotropic Medication Patterns among Youth in Foster Care." *Pediatrics* 121(1):157–163.

INDEX